The Audiogram Workbook

Audiometric Symbols And Abbreviations

Audiogram Legend[1]

		R	L
AIR	Unmasked	○	X
	Masked	△	☐
BONE	Unmasked	<	>
	Masked	[	]
SOUND FIELD		S	S
AIDED		A	A
NO RESPONSE		↙	↘

Descriptive Boundaries[2] for Hearing Threshold Status

0-20 dB HL	Normal range-Adults
21-25 dB HL	Slight
26-40 dB HL	Mild
41-55 dB HL	Moderate
56-70 dB HL	Moderately Severe
71-90 dB HL	Severe
91 dB+	Profound

Audiometric Abbreviations

A/B	Air conduction-bone conduction (as in air-bone gap)
AC	Air conduction
BC	Bone conduction
CNT	Could not test
COMP	Compliance
DNT	Did not test
dB	Decibel
HL	Hearing level. Used also for hearing loss.
Hz	Hertz or cycles per second
MEP	Middle ear pressure
PV	Physical volume
SN	Sensori-neural
SRT	Speech recognition threshold
SDS	Speech discrimination score
WDS	Word discrimination score (same as SDS)
WNL	Within normal limits

---

[1]Adapted from American Speech-Language-Hearing Association (1990), Guidelines for Audiometric Symbols, Asha, April 1990 (Supplement 2), pp. 25-30.

[2]Adapted from Davis, H. Guide for the Classification and Evaluation of Hearing Handicap, Trans Amer Acad Otolaryng, 1965, pp. 740-751.

The Audiogram Workbook

Sharon T. Hepfner
Division of Audiology
Department of Otolaryngology
University of Cincinatti
Cincinatti, Ohio

1998

Thieme
New York • Stuttgart

Thieme Medical Publishers, Inc.
381 Park Avenue South
New York, NY 10016

The Audiogram Workbook
Sharon T. Hepfner

Important note: Medical knowledge is ever-changing. As new research and clinical experience broaden our knowledge, changes in treatment and drug therapy may be required. The authors and editors of the material herein have consulted sources believed to be reliable in their efforts to provide information that is complete and in accord with the standards accepted at the time of publication. However, in view of the possibility of human error by the authors, editors, or publisher of the work herein, or changes in medical knowledge, neither the authors, editors, publisher, nor any other party who has been involved in the preparation of this work, warrants that the information contained herein is in every respect accurate or complete, and they are not responsible for any errors or omissions or for the results obtained from use of such information. Readers are encouraged to confirm the information contained herein with other sources. For example, readers are advised to check the product information sheet included in the package of each drug they plan to administer to be certain that the information contained in this publication is accurate and that changes have not been made in the recommended dose or in the contraindications for administration. This recommendation is of particular importance in connection with new or infrequently used drugs.

Some of the product names, patents, and registered designs referred to in this book are in fact registered trademarks or proprietary names even though specific reference to this fact is not always made in the text. Therefore, the appearance of a name without designation as proprietary is not to be construed as a representation by the publisher that it is in the public domain.

Printed in the United States of America

5 4 3 2 1

TNY ISBN 0-86577-719-5
GTV ISBN 3-13-109761-2

To Norma T. Hopkinson

Preface

The Audiogram Workbook was prepared in response to specific requests from ENT residents and from audiologists new to the medical setting. They have asked for illustrative cases that will assist them in recognizing and interpreting the patterns and variations within the standard audiologic test battery.

It is said that clinical intuition cannot be taught. However, the successful clinician can, from experience, develop the ability to recognize and appreciate the significance of the nuances in the test results when considered together with the patient's symptoms and behavior. The importance of being able to move beyond the abstractions of traditional classroom/textbook examples to consider the uniqueness of each patient cannot be underestimated.

During 27 years of clinical supervision and instruction, I have recognized the need for an effective self-administered training tool with multiple honest clinical examples. The workbook format was the logical solution. The old medical school axiom, "see one, do one, teach one," does not apply here! Included in The Audiogram Workbook are 135 cases for practical assessment and professional development.

This workbook provides advanced students of audiology and otology practice in interpretation and reporting of audiometric test results. It also affords an opportunity to appreciate a wide variety of etiologies and their manifestations under the broad categories of auditory disorders. Commonly used medical and audiological abbreviations have been included to facilitate chart and report review.

All of the audiograms in this collection are actual, unabridged tests performed on adults in busy ENT practices and clinics. Some patients were tested at their hospital bedside or in intensive care units. These settings naturally have time constraints for testing and interpretation. There is also the additional challenge imposed by a patient's mental or physical state.

The otologist and audiologist work "hand-in-glove" in the assessment of patients with ear, hearing, and/or vestibular complaints. Both are responsible for efficient, accurate diagnosis. Only when each discipline speaks the other's language fluently, is this possible. It is hoped that the information contained herein will facilitate the understanding of the audiological contribution to the differential diagnosis of otologic pathologies.

The reader is invited to evaluate (and critique) the following audiograms and then compare his or her own interpretation with the original report. The presenting information that precedes each case is that which was available to, or deduced by, the audiologist prior to testing.

It seems appropriate that an audiogram workbook describe how those tests were accomplished. The first section of this book suggests basic test instructions followed by many of the procedural modifications imposed by unusual patient conditions and situations. They are presented as suggestions intended to optimize audiologic testing at the level of clinician-patient interaction.

Contents

Foundations For Accurate Assessment

Clinician-Patient Interaction 3

Preparation for Testing 3

Basic Test Instructions 3
    Basic Instructions for Alert, Oriented, English Speaking Patients 3
    Speech Recognition Threshold (SRT) 3
    Word Recognition Test (Speech Discrimination) 4
    Pure Tone Air Conduction Tests 4
    The Weber 4
    Pure Tone Bone Conduction Test 5
    Pure Tone or Speech Stenger Test 5

Patient Conditions and Circumstances Requiring Procedure Modifications 6
    Modified Instructions for Non-English Speaking Patients 6
    Accents, Dialects, Speech Disorders 6
    Tracheostomies and Laryngectomies 6
    Otorrhea 6
    Burns and Open Wounds 7
    Hospital Patients at Bedside 7
    Uncooperative Patients 8
    Mentally Ill Patients 8
    Prisoners 9
    Patients with Communicable Diseases 9

Reporting Test Results 9

AUDIOGRAM SECTION 1   Sensori-Neural Hearing Loss 11
AUDIOGRAM SECTION 2   Conductive Hearing Loss 123
AUDIOGRAM SECTION 3   Mixed Hearing Loss 165
AUDIOGRAM SECTION 4   Normal Hearing 217
AUDIOGRAM SECTION 5   Nonorganic Hearing Loss 239
AUDIOGRAM SECTION 6   Practice Audiograms 251

Glossary of Commonly Used Medical Abbreviations 269

Suggested Readings 279

The Audiogram Workbook

FOUNDATIONS FOR ACCURATE ASSESSMENT

CLINICIAN-PATIENT INTERACTION

The audiologist is the link between the equipment and the patient. The skill with which the testing is performed will be the decisive difference between audiometric results that are meaningful and those that are diagnostically misleading. The reliability of the test results can be adversely affected by equipment malfunction, position and pressure of the earphones or bone-conduction oscillator, patient discomfort, the conditions of the test environment, and ambiguous test instructions.

As is the case with any clinician, the audiologist's experience, insight, and personality affect the patient's behavior and, eventually, the test results and their interpretation.

PREPARATION FOR TESTING

1. Ensure cords are firmly plugged in. (Cleaning crews may have dislodged them.) Also, check cords after testing an agitated patient.

2. Perform daily listening checks on all equipment.

3. Check impedance probes for obstructions.

BASIC TEST INSTRUCTIONS

Basic Instructions for Alert, Oriented, English Speaking Patients

The patient is seated at a modest angle which will allow the clinician to observe his or her face and hands. Having established which is the (better) ear that will be tested first, the audiologist gives the following instructions for speech audiometry (only!), places the earphones on the patient, and proceeds to the equipment.

Speech Recognition Threshold (SRT)

"You will be asked to repeat some easy words that we say every day, words like baseball, airplane, or mailman. Please repeat the test words. Some of them are very,very soft, and you will have to guess. That's OK, that is supposed to happen. Remember, repeat the words, and take a guess when you need to."

With the SRT test completed, the presentation level is adjusted to the discrimination test level, and the following instructions are given:

Word Recognition Test (Speech Discrimination)

"You did well. This is easier to hear, isn't it? Now you need to repeat some more words. They will not be any softer than this. Remember to take a guess if you are not sure what the word is."

Suggestion

Some people are confused by the carrying phrase used for these word tests. They may repeat the phrase but not the test word. In that case, the tests must be presented by live voice with the phrase omitted.

Suggestion

If the patient's discrimination scores are reduced for each ear, present the test binaurally. This third score may help differentiate between peripheral and central dysfunction and will also provide information necessary for hearing aid selection.

Pure Tone Air Conduction Tests

"Now, in this part of the test, you will be listening for some very soft beeping tones coming into your right (left) earphone. They will sound like beep, beep, beep.

Listen carefully for the first tone beeps and push your "yes" button as soon as you hear them start. Remember, it is important that we know when you are first begining to hear the tone beeps so be ready to push this button as soon as you hear them start."

Suggestion

If the patient is confused by the use of the response button, take it from him or her and tell the patient to just say "yes" when he or she hears the tones. (A hand-raise response is not always satisfactory because the movement may be slight or hesitant.)

The Weber

Activate a steady tone through the oscillator at the frequency where you suspect there will be the clearest indication of localization. Use at least a 50 dB intensity.

"I am going to hold this against your forehead. You will hear a tone somewhere in your head. There is no right or wrong answer. Just tell me where the tone seems to go first."

Suggestion

Test at several frequencies. Vary the intensity if the patient's responses are vague. Watch the patient for eye shifts when the oscillator is first applied to his or her head. Many people are reluctant to admit that the tone was heard in their "bad" ear.

Pure Tone Bone Conduction Test

"I am going to put this behind your right (left) ear. Now we need to put this earphone over your other ear. The soft beeping tones are going to be in your uncovered ear. Please push the button when you begin to hear the soft beeping sounds. Now, in your other ear, there will be a wooshing sound that is there on purpose to keep that ear from helping to hear. Please listen only in the open ear for beeping...that is the only thing that is important for us to know about."

(Touch the test ear for reinforcement.)

Suggestion

It is very disconcerting to most people to have the masking noise turned off and on as the clinician records the threshold levels. For some people, the bone conduction headband and oscillator are very uncomfortable. Sympathize with them, and complete the test as rapidly as possible.

Pure Tone or Speech Stenger Test

To validate a unilateral hearing loss, the Stenger is the test of choice. Some clinicians perform this test with no additional instructions. This can be accomplished after establishing speech or pure tone thresholds in the usual manner. The audiometer is prepared for simultaneous presentation of identical information. The level at which the better ear is set is usually 10 dB above threshold, and the poor ear is set 10 to 15 dB below admitted threshold. If a response is obtained, it is a true loss. If no response is given, it means that the patient has heard in the poorer ear. Lower the level of the signal to the poor ear in 5 dB steps until the patient responds. The lowest level at which no response was obtained will be close to threshold.

PATIENT CONDITIONS AND CIRCUMSTANCES REQUIRING PROCEDURE MODIFICATIONS

Modified Instructions for Non-English Speaking Patients

Speech Testing: Many people who have been living in the United States for a few months are familiar with some of the spondee words such as "airplane," "hotdog," baseball" etc. Begin by holding the earphones in your hand as an indication that you are preparing to test the patient. Say the word "baseball" as you point to your mouth. Point to the patient's mouth and look at him or her expectently. Try several words and say "OK" or "good", with a smile, when they repeat the word. Using selected spondees, you should be able to obtain a good estimation of threshold.

Mark the speech section of the audiogram "SRT - selected words."

One can attempt to use live voice presentation of the word discrimination lists. No carrying phrase is used in this case. If the person tries to repeat phonetically, you may get some indication about any marked difference between ears. Star (*) the scoring section on the audiogram, and explain your observation in the report.

Pure Tone Test instructions are easily pantomimed and should not be difficult for the patient to understand. It is usually more efficient to conduct these tests face-to-face.

Accents, Dialects, Speech Disorders

If scoring the word recognition/ discrimination test responses is affected by the patient's articulation, accent or dialect, ask that the patient spell the word that he or she just repeated. If the patient is unable to do so, then the final test score must be labled as "approximate" on the face of the test sheet. The report should then state that the scoring was contaminated by the patient's speech, or that "English is not the patient's basic language and responses were subject to interpretation."

Tracheostomies and Laryngectomies

If the patient is alert and is used to covering the tracheostomy for speaking, there should not be any significant problem in obtaining speech scores. The rate of presentation may have to be adjusted.

Patients who use an artificial larynx or esophageal speech can be reliably scored. However, if their oral communication is labored or unclear, they can be asked to write their answers on a numbered tablet.

Otorrhea

Copius discharge from the middle ear or a cerebral spinal fluid leak pools in the concha and seems to increase with earphone pressure. The earphone must be covered to protect it and the patient from contamination. Use an earphone protector and one or two 4 X 4 gauze squares and have the patient hold the phone in a way that will reduce the pressure. Note on the audiogram that the earphone had to be manipulated because of the condition of the ear.

The audiologist wears gloves and disinfects the headset following the test. Impedance audiometry is not conducted on these ears.

Burns and Open Wounds

The first consideration is the patient's welfare. His or her wounds must be protected from contamination from the equipment. The protocal of scrub, gown, mask, and gloves is followed for bedside tests on burn victims. Prepare for testing any patient with fresh or open head wounds by disinfecting the earphones and cords and having on hand sterile 4 X 4's. Opening the 4 X 4's produces rectangular drapes that are placed across the top of the head, ear to ear. Extra pads over stapled areas may be required. Of course, the ear cushions are also covered.

Depending on the area of injury and the condition of the patient, it may be necessary to manipulate the audiometer with one hand and hold the earphone to the patient's head, with the other. This is also a necessary maneuver for patients with neck injuries supported by a halo, and for those with recent facial bone fractures or trauma to the pinna. Many standard test procedures will have to be modified. The test may also be taking place in a noisy environment.

The referring physicians need to have, at the very least, a gross estimate of the extent and nature (i.e., conductive or sensori-neural) of this person's hearing loss. This should be possible if the clinician is not attached to rigid test protocols.

Hospital Patients at Bedside

Go prepared, i.e., equipment, supplies, test forms, otoscope, etc. (Quite a few of these patients have had only cursory ear inspections and do indeed have excessive cerumen, narrowed ear canals, etc.)

Determine, by reading the orders in the patient's chart, why a hearing evaluation is being requested. Frequently, the patient's medical treatment involves medication known to be ototoxic. Some will be receiving experimental medications, and a baseline is required. Others have a long-standing loss, no hearing aid, and the hospital staff is having difficulty communicating with them. The clinician must make certain that the test summary and recommendations address the house staff's questions and concerns about their patient.

When testing any patient at bedside his or her condition is the first concern. The test environment is the second problem. That includes not only the noise and interruptions but the not-so-small difficulty of where to place the test equipment (portable audiometer, tympanometer and test forms).

If the patient has an SRT of greater than 30 dB in each ear, it is possible to do live voice speech testing. If there is any electronic medical equipment pumping or gurgling, the pure tone thresholds below 1000 Hz will have no value (unless the patient has a moderate low-to-mid frequency loss in each ear). You can obtain fairly reliable pure tone and bone conduction thresholds at 1KHz and above for a person with normal or mildly reduced thresholds — if that person is alert, cooperative, and motivated. The audiologist, in the meantime, is being composed and creative. For example, it may be possible for the patient's nurse to pull the plug on some of the equipment for enough time to permit a rapid scan for thresholds. Or, a patient can be assisted in focusing on the test ear by having a low level of broad-band masking noise in the opposite ear.

Patients who are very ill and/or heavily medicated have a difficult time staying awake for the test and will require frequent efforts to waken them and reinstruct. Sometimes you can obtain reponses to pure tone stimuli by holding their hand and requesting that they squeeze when they hear.

It is often best to leave a chart note stating that the patient could not be aroused and that audiology is to be contacted again when the condition improves. An ABR test may also be an option (especially for head injuries where one must rule out severe hearing loss as the cause for the lack of response).

Uncooperative Patients

About 4% of a clinic population can be expected to have a functional overlay on their test results. People seeking SSI disability or other financial compensation are the most common sources of functional problems. However, the examiner should be particularly alert when hearing complaints have vague origins. There are also some mannerisms that are apparent to the experienced examiner. These may include an obvious avoidance of eye contact with the examiner, facial grimaces with an exaggerated listening posture, and half word responses to spondee word presentations. Probably the most sensitive indicator of functional loss is a pure tone/word recognition discrepancy of 15 dB or more.

In cases of unilateral exaggeration, the Stenger Test is very helpful. In a time-restricted situation, it is most efficient to complete the objective tympanogram and acoustic reflex threshold tests first. Sometimes it is better to go ahead and record the speech and pure tone thresholds that the patient will admit to and point out the inter and intra test discrepancies in the report. Identify those test results that appear to be the best indicators of the organic level of hearing. Schedule a retest in not less than 3 weeks. If there is another audiologist available, have him or her conduct the retest.

Mentally Ill Patients

Many patients with serious psychiatric problems are referred because they "hear voices." Often these are lonely, elderly people with unaided severe hearing loss. Fitting these people with hearing aids can bring about a marked improvement in their mental state. Other patients are being referred because their hearing loss is impeding therapy.

There might be some testing problems with those who are heavily medicated. Behaviors vary. Some sit slumped over and are unresponsive. They require frequent encouragement and reinstruction. Others can be very agitated — undressing, getting up from the chair, taking off the earphones, pulling at the cords. The clinician must use a firm, authoritarian voice to establish control. A very few patients are potentially dangerous, and their attendant will stay with them in the test booth. Do not wear a nametag.

Prisoners

The audiologist is not going to know, and does not have to know, why this patient is handcuffed and shackled. Prisoners are accompanied by deputies, and these prisoners are not going anywhere they should not. If you see that they are accompanied by two deputies, remove your nametag. Do not leave ballpoint pens or cerumen picks, etc., within their reach. Their hearing complaints are the same as the unincarcerated population. Their histories most typically are of chronic ear disease, blows to the head, and noise exposure. In terms of auditory rehabilitation, it is difficult to arrange for hearing aids for them while they are in jail. The Bureau of Vocational Rehabilitation (BVR) can, and will, help.

Patients with Communicable Diseases

To prevent embarrassing any patient by singling him or her out for special precautions, it is wise to begin the day with a mask loose around your neck and ready to use. Boxes of gloves and antiseptic wipes or solutions are already at hand in each test area. The use of any or all of these forms of protection should appear to the patient to be an ordinary procedure. Clinics and hospitals have protocals for protection and decontamination for airborne diseases.

A patient with a compromised immune system or fresh wounds should be protected from any infection or virus that the clinician is experiencing. The clinician must wear gloves.

Both patient and clinician wear masks.

REPORTING TEST RESULTS

Reports should be concise and written in a manner that allows the physician or referral source quick access to pertinent information. Unusual findings or matters of concern should be highlighted.

SECTION 1
SENSORI-NEURAL HEARING LOSS

PRESENTING INFORMATION

Strong family hx of progressing hearing loss. Severe impairment by age 9 in this case as well as other family members. She wears a high power BTE hearing aid on left ear (only) which provides only enhanced voice awareness. Her speech reflects the hearing impairment. She depends on visual cues to supplement amplification.

Middle ear compliance and pressure are WNL, AU. The acoustic reflex is not elicited AU.

Pt. Information:

M _____ F _X_ Age: _37_

SPEECH AUDIOMETRY

	SRT		WORD RECOGNITION		
	dB	Mask	%	Mask	SL
RIGHT	75		16		30
LEFT	75		0		30
RIGHT					
LEFT					
BIN					

MASKING LEVELS USED

In Right (testing left)	AIR								
	BONE								
In Left (testing right)	AIR								
	BONE								
WEBER Lateralizes To									
		250	500	750	1000	1500	2000	3000	4000	6000	8000

PURE-TONE AUDIOGRAM
FREQUENCY IN HERTZ (Hz)

EVALUATION _____

_____

_____

_____

_____

_____

_____

_____

_____

_____

_____

_____

_____

_____

INTERPRETATION

Bilateral SN hearing loss characterized by a moderate, steeply sloping to severe loss through the low to mid frequencies. The impairment is profound above 1000 Hz, right ear, and above 750 Hz, left ear. There is poor or no speech discrimination ability. Middle ear compliance and pressure are WNL. There is no acoustic reflex elicited AU. Results are consistent with hx of familial hearing loss.

RECOMMENDATIONS

Evaluation with binaural amplification and assistive listening devices. Provide information re cochlear implant. Provide literature re availability and importance of genetic counseling.

PRESENTING INFORMATION

Recently noticed deterioration in right ear hearing sensitivity. No vestibular complaints. Cannot use right ear on telephone for past few weeks. Reports "strange twitching sensation" on right side of face.

Middle ear function is normal AU. The acoustic reflex is absent, AD, and present, AS.

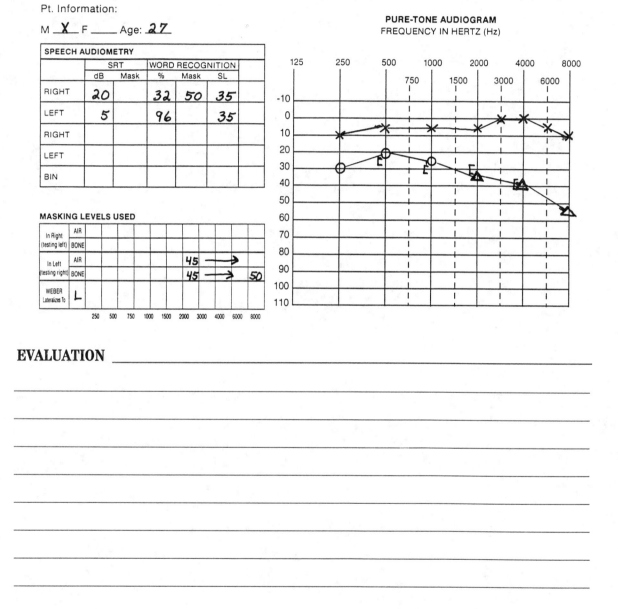

Pt. Information:

M **X** F ____ Age: **27**

PURE-TONE AUDIOGRAM
FREQUENCY IN HERTZ (Hz)

SPEECH AUDIOMETRY

	SRT		WORD RECOGNITION		
	dB	Mask	%	Mask	SL
RIGHT	20		32	50	35
LEFT	5		96		35
RIGHT					
LEFT					
BIN					

MASKING LEVELS USED

In Right (testing left)	AIR									
	BONE									
In Left (testing right)	AIR				45 →					
	BONE				45 →		50			
WEBER Lateralizes To	L									

250 500 750 1000 1500 2000 3000 4000 6000 8000

EVALUATION _____

INTERPRETATION

Normal hearing sensitivity, word discrimination ability, middle ear function, and acoustic reflex activity in the left ear. Mild-to-moderate SN loss with poor speech discrimination, right ear. Considering that middle ear compliance and pressure are WNL, AU, the fact that the acoustic reflex is absent with right ipsilateral and left contralateral presentation is significant. R/O right retrocochlear pathology.

RECOMMENDATION

Evaluation for site of lesion.

OUTCOME

A 1.0 cm by 1.2 cm by 1.3 cm mass (consistent with acoustic neuroma) was identified at the right cerebellopontine angle also involving the intracanalicular portion of right VII and VIII nerve complex.

PRESENTING INFORMATION

Gradual onset of bilateral hearing loss. Mild tinnitus - not localized. No vestibular problems. Otologic exam identified "cherry red" left TM. Normal tympanograms. The acoustic reflex is present in the right ear and is absent in the left ear.

Pt. Information:

M _____ F _X_ Age: _76_

SPEECH AUDIOMETRY

	SRT		WORD RECOGNITION		
	dB	Mask	%	Mask	SL
RIGHT	25		100		30
LEFT	30		100		30
RIGHT			88	70	55
LEFT			92	70	55
BIN					

MASKING LEVELS USED

In Right (testing left)	AIR									
	BONE									
In Left (testing right)	AIR									
	BONE									
WEBER Lateralizes To	NO	—		—						

250 500 750 1000 1500 2000 3000 4000 6000 8000

PURE-TONE AUDIOGRAM
FREQUENCY IN HERTZ (Hz)

EVALUATION

_____

_____

_____

_____

_____

_____

_____

_____

_____

_____

_____

_____

_____

_____

_____

_____

INTERPRETATION

Bilateral (symmetrical) mild, sloping to moderately severe, SN hearing loss. Speech discrimination ability is excellent. Symmetrical, nonsignificant PI-PB rollover test results. Weber does not lateralize, and the tympanogram for each ear is WNL. The acoustic reflex is present (without decay) in the right ear and is absent in the left ear. The acoustic reflex is the only clear finding that implicates the left ear.

OUTCOME

Left glomus jugulare tumor confirmed by MRI.

PRESENTING INFORMATION

Progressing hearing loss. Normal tympanograms with reflex in each ear. Hx of exposure to gunfire (large weapons) during military service. Family hx of hearing loss (all siblings). No significant health problems.

Normal middle ear function AU. Acoustic reflex present AU.

Pt. Information:

M __X__ F _____ Age: __44__

SPEECH AUDIOMETRY

	SRT dB	SRT Mask	WORD RECOGNITION %	WORD RECOGNITION Mask	WORD RECOGNITION SL	
RIGHT	35		68		35	
LEFT	40		76		35	
RIGHT			88		45	
LEFT						
BIN						

MASKING LEVELS USED

In Right (testing left)	AIR									
	BONE									
In Left (testing right)	AIR									
	BONE									
WEBER Lateralizes To										
		250	500	750	1000	1500	2000	3000	4000	6000	8000

PURE-TONE AUDIOGRAM
FREQUENCY IN HERTZ (Hz)

EVALUATION

_____

_____

_____

_____

_____

_____

_____

_____

_____

_____

_____

_____

_____

_____

_____

INTERPRETATION

Bilateral mild-to-severe SN hearing loss characterized by mid-frequency notch. Speech discrimination ability is fair-good (improves with presentation level). Normal middle ear compliance and pressure AU. The acoustic reflex is elicited AU.

RECOMMENDATIONS

Hearing aid evaluation. Binaural amplification is indicated. The pt. has been provided with literature re hearing loss which includes a discussion of familial hearing loss. Annual retests have been recommended.

PRESENTING INFORMATION

Widely fluctuating hearing levels and word discrimination ability. Has been followed and treated for syphilis (for 6 years). Difficult to test due to many false positive responses.

Normal tympanograms. The acoustic reflex is present in the right ear and is absent in the left ear.

Pt. Information:

M _____ F _X_ Age: _63_

SPEECH AUDIOMETRY

	SRT		WORD RECOGNITION		
	dB	Mask	%	Mask	SL
RIGHT	35		92		30
LEFT	50		56	60	30
RIGHT					
LEFT					
BIN					

MASKING LEVELS USED

		250	500	750	1000	1500	2000	3000	4000	6000	8000
In Right (testing left)	AIR	60	60								
	BONE		65	60	65	60		70		70	
In Left (testing right)	AIR										
	BONE										
WEBER Lateralizes To											

PURE-TONE AUDIOGRAM
FREQUENCY IN HERTZ (Hz)

EVALUATION

_____

_____

_____

_____

_____

_____

_____

_____

_____

_____

_____

_____

_____

_____

INTERPRETATION

RIGHT EAR: Mild-to-severe SN hearing loss with good speech discrimination ability. Normal tympanogram. Normal acoustic reflex activity.

LEFT EAR: Moderately severe to severe SN loss with a very reduced speech discrimination score. Normal tympanogram. The acoustic reflex is absent in this ear.

RECOMMENDATIONS

Refer for assistive hearing devices. (Conventional hearing aids would be difficult to fit because her loss fluctuates from mild to severe, and word recognition scores in either ear have frequently been below 20%.) Hearing status should continue to be monitored twice a year or PRN.

PRESENTING INFORMATION

Teenager with progressing hearing loss. Complains of being unable to use left ear on telephone. Frequent severe headaches. He appeared to be somewhat disoriented and had some difficulty focusing on the tasks involved in the hearing exam. There is radiographic evidence of bilateral acoustic neuromas. There is no known family hx of neurofibromatosis.

Normal tympanograms and absence of acoustic reflex AU.

Pt. Information:

M __X__ F _____ Age: __18__

SPEECH AUDIOMETRY

	SRT dB	SRT Mask	WORD RECOGNITION %	WORD RECOGNITION Mask	WORD RECOGNITION SL
RIGHT	35		100		30
LEFT	45		16	60	30
RIGHT					
LEFT					
BIN					

PURE-TONE AUDIOGRAM
FREQUENCY IN HERTZ (Hz)

MASKING LEVELS USED

		250	500	750	1000	1500	2000	3000	4000	6000	8000
In Right (testing left)	AIR					80					
	BONE		70	65	80	60					
In Left (testing right)	AIR										
	BONE		70	65		60					
WEBER Lateralizes To											

EVALUATION

INTERPRETATION

RIGHT EAR: Mild-moderate SN hearing loss with excellent word discrimination.

LEFT EAR: Mild-to-severe SN loss with very poor word discrimination. Both ears have normal middle ear compliance and pressure. The acoustic reflex is absent AU.

Note: Inconsistent responses. Fair reliability.

OUTCOME

Surgical removal of bilateral acoustic tumors is planned. Audiology will monitor patient's communication needs. Arrangements for home schooling and sign language classes have been made.

PRESENTING INFORMATION

Pt. states that the hearing loss has been present since infancy and has been attributed to scarlet fever at age 3 months. Wearing hearing aid on the right ear. Oral communication. Good lipreading skills.

Normal tympanogram AU. No acoustic reflex.

Pt. Information:

M __X__ F _____ Age: _56_

SPEECH AUDIOMETRY

	SRT		WORD RECOGNITION		
	dB	Mask	%	Mask	SL
RIGHT	80		52		35
LEFT	NR		CNE		
RIGHT					
LEFT					
BIN					

MASKING LEVELS USED

In Right (testing left)	AIR	95								
	BONE									
In Left (testing right)	AIR									
	BONE									
WEBER Lateralizes To										
		250	500	750	1000	1500	2000	3000	4000	6000	8000

PURE-TONE AUDIOGRAM
FREQUENCY IN HERTZ (Hz)

EVALUATION _____

_____

_____

_____

_____

_____

_____

_____

_____

_____

_____

_____

_____

INTERPRETATION

RIGHT EAR: Severe-to-profound SN hearing loss with reduced word recognition consistent with the degree and nature of the loss.

LEFT EAR: Profound SN hearing loss with no response to speech testing. There is normal middle ear pressure and compliance AU. The acoustic reflex is not elicited AU.

RECOMMENDATION

This pt. is aware of assistive devices and sources. He is seeking Social Security Disability status (SSI) and has declined referral to the Bureau of Vocational Rehabilitation (BVR).

PRESENTING INFORMATION

Hx of right cholesteatoma for which he underwent surgery 2 years ago. Since the surgery, he has had a profound right ear hearing loss with episodes of recurrent discharge and occasional pain. His cc is primarily positional vertigo.

Right tympanogram deferred. Left tympanogram is WNL.

Pt. Information:

M __X__ F _____ Age: **60**

SPEECH AUDIOMETRY

	SRT dB	SRT Mask	WORD RECOGNITION %	WORD RECOGNITION Mask	WORD RECOGNITION SL
RIGHT	NR	75			
LEFT	20		88		30
RIGHT					
LEFT					
BIN					

MASKING LEVELS USED

		250	500	750	1000	1500	2000	3000	4000	6000	8000
In Right (testing left)	AIR										
	BONE										
In Left (testing right)	AIR	80 →						95			
	BONE		80 →					95			
WEBER Lateralizes To											

PURE-TONE AUDIOGRAM
FREQUENCY IN HERTZ (Hz)

EVALUATION

_____

_____

_____

_____

_____

_____

_____

_____

_____

_____

_____

_____

_____

_____

INTERPRETATION

RIGHT EAR: Profound SN loss with no measurable hearing for speech. The Pure Tone Stenger Test results are negative and support the severity of the loss. Tympanometry was deferred due to the condition of the ear.

LEFT EAR: Borderline-normal low and mid frequency sensitivity with a precipitous drop to a profound SN loss above 2000 Hz. Speech discrimination is good. The tympanogram is WNL.

RECOMMENDATIONS

An ENG and radiologic evaluation have been scheduled re his vertigo.

A hearing aid evaluation and trial with a BICROS instrument is suggested.

PRESENTING INFORMATION:

Hearing impairment attributed to years of unprotected noise exposure, and, very recently, severe head trauma suffered in a vehicular accident. His face and head wounds are partially healed; the right TM perforation has closed.

Normal middle ear pressure AU. Hypercompliant TM, AD. The acoustic reflex is absent AU.

Pt. Information:

M __X__ F _____ Age: _71_

PURE-TONE AUDIOGRAM
FREQUENCY IN HERTZ (Hz)

SPEECH AUDIOMETRY

	SRT		WORD RECOGNITION		
	dB	Mask	%	Mask	SL
RIGHT	30		40		30
LEFT	30		44		30
RIGHT			40	60	40
LEFT			72	60	40
BIN					

MASKING LEVELS USED

In Right (testing left)	AIR									
	BONE									
In Left (testing right)	AIR									
	BONE									
WEBER Lateralizes To										

EVALUATION _____

_____

_____

_____

_____

_____

_____

_____

_____

_____

_____

_____

_____

_____

INTERPRETATION

Bilateral steeply sloping (mild to severe) SN hearing loss. Speech discrimination scores are significantly reduced. The left ear score improves to "fair" with an increase in the test presentation level. Tympanometry reveals normal middle ear pressure AU. There is tympanometric evidence of hypercompliance of the right ear system but left ear compliance is WNL. The right ear results are consistent with the recently healed TM perforation. The ipsilateral acoustic reflex is absent AU.

RECOMMENDATION

A hearing aid evaluation should be considered for him upon completion of medical management and when medical clearance for hearing aid use can be given.

PRESENTING INFORMATION

The pt. sustained 55% total body surface burns in an explosion 3 months prior to this test. He had undergone extensive surgery/therapy. He regained full consciousness less than a week ago and complains of right ear fullness with hearing loss. Aminoglycoside Rx for infection control.

Testing was accomplished with sterile gauze draped over his head and padding the ears. The bone conduction oscillator was hand-held. Tympanometry was not attempted. In spite of his discomfort and the ambient noise from life-support equipment, the results appear to provide reliable indications of his hearing status.

Pt. Information:

M __X__ F _____ Age: __35__

PURE-TONE AUDIOGRAM
FREQUENCY IN HERTZ (Hz)

SPEECH AUDIOMETRY

	SRT		WORD RECOGNITION		
	dB	Mask	%	Mask	SL
RIGHT	5		92		30
LEFT	5		88		30
RIGHT					
LEFT					
BIN					

MASKING LEVELS USED

In Right (testing left)	AIR									65
	BONE									
In Left (testing right)	AIR									
	BONE									
WEBER Lateralizes To										

250 500 750 1000 1500 2000 3000 4000 6000 8000

EVALUATION

_____

INTERPRETATION

Bilateral normal hearing sensitivity 250 through 4000 Hz. There is a mild, high frequency deficit in the right ear and a precipitous, mild to severe, high frequency SN loss in the left ear. Speech discrimination scores are fairly good AU. The condition of the pt.'s ears and ear canals prevents middle ear measurements.

RECOMMENDATION

Weekly monitoring of hearing status.

PRESENTING INFORMATION:

This 37-year-old woman complains of years of difficulty hearing and understanding speech. She has been advised that her hearing test results are "normal." Recently, increased difficulty hearing conversational speech has led her to seek another opinion.

Normal tympanograms. Normal acoustic reflex thresholds. No reflex decay AU.

Pt. Information:

M _____ F _X_ Age: _37_

SPEECH AUDIOMETRY

	SRT dB	SRT Mask	WORD RECOGNITION %	WORD RECOGNITION Mask	WORD RECOGNITION SL
RIGHT	10		84	35	40
LEFT	0		100		35
RIGHT			56	55	75
LEFT			100		80
BIN					

MASKING LEVELS USED

		250	500	750	1000	1500	2000	3000	4000	6000	8000
In Right (testing left)	AIR										
	BONE										
In Left (testing right)	AIR										
	BONE	45			45	50					
WEBER Lateralizes To											

PURE-TONE AUDIOGRAM
FREQUENCY IN HERTZ (Hz)

EVALUATION _____

_____

_____

_____

_____

_____

_____

_____

_____

_____

_____

_____

INTERPRETATION

RIGHT EAR: Results reflect a mild high frequency and 250 Hz SN hearing loss. The speech discrimination score is fairly good, but there is significant PI-PB rollover. The tympanogram is normal, acoustic reflex thresholds are normal, and there is no reflex decay.

LEFT EAR: Hearing sensitivity, speech discrimination ability, middle ear compliance and pressure, and acoustic reflex thresholds are normal. There is no acoustic reflex decay. There is no PI-PB rollover.

RECOMMENDATION

Refer for ABR testing due to asymmetry of the hearing loss and the positive finding for rollover.

OUTCOME

Normal ABR test results for each ear. The CT scan revealed proximal congenital stenosis of the internal auditory canals in their rostral to caudal dimensions. No focal enlargement to suggest acoustic neuroma.

PRESENTING INFORMATION

Sudden hearing loss, left ear. Started on steroids 2 weeks ago when the test of the left ear revealed a 70 dB average hearing threshold, and her speech discrimination score was 30%. She returns for follow-up reporting that her vertigo and tinnitus have lessened and that her hearing status is improving.

Pt. Information:

M _____ F _X_ Age: _35_

SPEECH AUDIOMETRY

	SRT		WORD RECOGNITION		
	dB	Mask	%	Mask	SL
RIGHT	5		96		30
LEFT	50	50	96	60	30
RIGHT					
LEFT					
BIN					

MASKING LEVELS USED

In Right (testing left)	AIR	60	→		65			
	BONE	60	→		65			
In Left (testing right)	AIR							
	BONE							
WEBER Lateralizes To								
		250	500	750	1000	1500	2000	3000 4000 6000 8000

PURE-TONE AUDIOGRAM
FREQUENCY IN HERTZ (Hz)

EVALUATION

INTERPRETATION

RIGHT EAR: Normal hearing thresholds with excellent speech discrimination ability. Normal tympanogram with acoustic reflex.

LEFT EAR: Moderate SN loss with excellent speech discrimination. Normal tympanogram with absent acoustic reflex. Left ear hearing thresholds have improved 20 dB, and speech discrimination has returned to normal following steroid Rx.

OUTCOME

MRI of brain was negative. Pt. did not return for further medical or audiological follow-up.

PRESENTING INFORMATION

Pt. complains of tinnitus and unsteadiness as well as some difficulty hearing. He assumed that his ears "needed a good cleaning."

Normal tympanograms. The acoustic reflex is absent AU.

Pt. Information:

M __X__ F _____ Age: __63__

SPEECH AUDIOMETRY

	SRT		WORD RECOGNITION		
	dB	Mask	%	Mask	SL
RIGHT	15		92		35
LEFT	30		76	45	35
RIGHT					
LEFT			50	65	65
BIN					

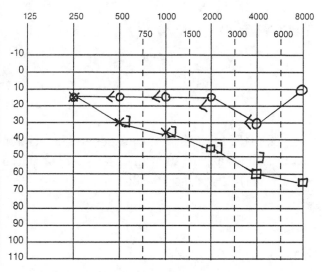

PURE-TONE AUDIOGRAM
FREQUENCY IN HERTZ (Hz)

MASKING LEVELS USED

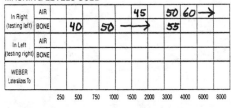

		250	500	750	1000	1500	2000	3000	4000	6000	8000
In Right (testing left)	AIR					45		50	60 →		
	BONE	40	50	→		55					
In Left (testing right)	AIR										
	BONE										
WEBER Lateralizes To											

EVALUATION

_____

_____

_____

_____

_____

_____

_____

_____

_____

_____

_____

_____

_____

_____

_____

_____

_____

INTERPRETATION

RIGHT EAR: Hearing sensitivity is within normal limits. His speech discrimination score is good. Middle ear pressure and compliance are normal. The acoustic reflex is absent.

LEFT EAR: A mild , sloping to severe, SN hearing loss and a reduced speech discrimination score. The tympanogram is normal, but the acoustic reflex is also absent in this ear. There is significant PI-PB rollover.

RECOMMENDATION

R/O retrocochlear lesion.

OUTCOME

The MRI of the brain revealed mild cerebellar atrophy. The ABR response for the left ear was abnormal and indicated retrocochlear pathology for that ear. (The right ABR results were WNL.) Pt. was lost to follow-up.

PRESENTING INFORMATION

Pt. was first evaluated 5 months ago for his complaint of fluctuating hearing loss. His lab workup was negative (including syphilis). His hearing test identified significant SN loss, AU, which was asymmetrical. His left ear speech discrimination score was poor. He returned for this continued evaluation 5 months later.

Normal middle ear function AU with no acoustic reflex.

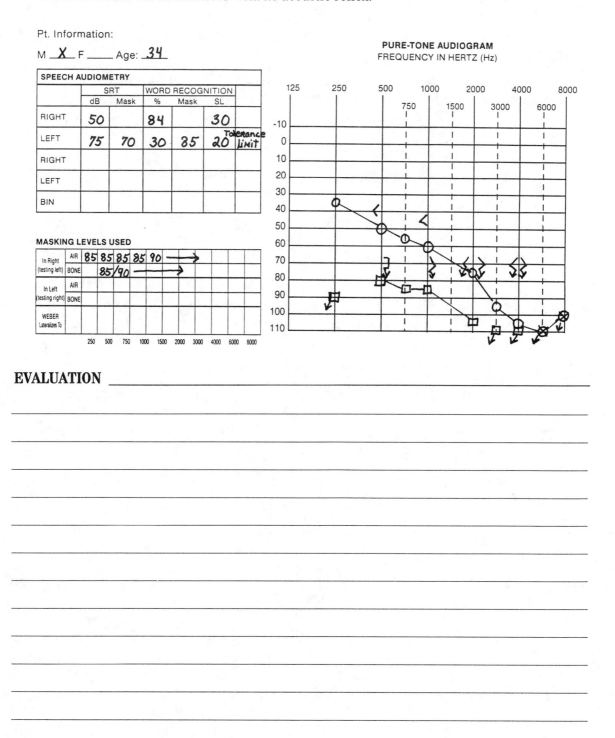

Pt. Information:

M __X__ F _____ Age: __34__

PURE-TONE AUDIOGRAM
FREQUENCY IN HERTZ (Hz)

SPEECH AUDIOMETRY

	SRT		WORD RECOGNITION			
	dB	Mask	%	Mask	SL	
RIGHT	50		84		30	
LEFT	75	70	30	85	20	Tolerance limit
RIGHT						
LEFT						
BIN						

MASKING LEVELS USED

In Right (testing left)	AIR	85	85	85	85	90	→		
	BONE		85/90		→			
In Left (testing right)	AIR							
	BONE							
WEBER Lateralizes To								

250 500 750 1000 1500 2000 3000 4000 6000 8000

EVALUATION _____

INTERPRETATION

RIGHT EAR: Stable, mild, sloping to profound, SN hearing loss. Fairly good speech discrimination score (stable). Normal tympanogram. Absent acoustic reflex.

LEFT EAR: Stable severe-to-profound SN hearing loss with the exception of an important increase in the loss at 250 Hz. Continues to have poor speech discrimination ability. Normal tympanogram. Absent acoustic reflex. Negative fistula test AU.

OUTCOME

CT scan of temporal bones was normal. Dx: Idiopathic SN hearing loss. Referred to a community speech and hearing center for amplification and assistive devices.

PRESENTING INFORMATION

Pt. was mugged by unknown assailants 2 days prior to this test. His injuries include fronto-parietal scalp lacerations and a concussion. Dried blood is present in, but does not occlude, each ear canal.

Normal right tympanogram; acoustic reflex is not elicited. Reduced middle ear compliance and absent reflex, left ear.

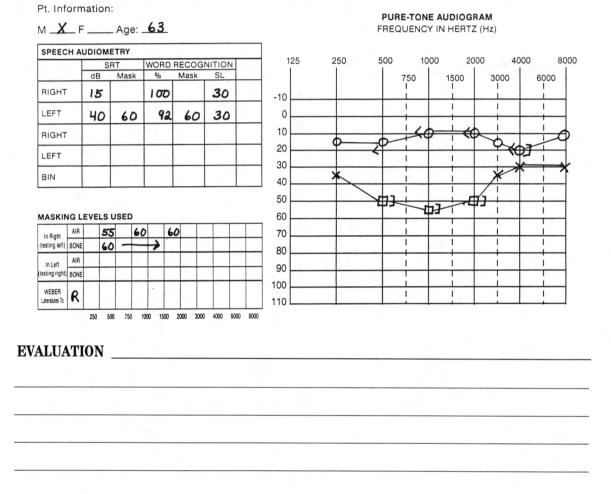

Pt. Information:

M __X__ F _____ Age: __63__

SPEECH AUDIOMETRY

	SRT		WORD RECOGNITION			
	dB	Mask	%	Mask	SL	
RIGHT	15		100		30	
LEFT	40	60	92	60	30	
RIGHT						
LEFT						
BIN						

MASKING LEVELS USED

In Right (testing left)	AIR	55		60		60			
	BONE	60	→						
In Left (testing right)	AIR								
	BONE								
WEBER Lateralizes To	R								

250 500 750 1000 1500 2000 3000 4000 6000 8000

PURE-TONE AUDIOGRAM
FREQUENCY IN HERTZ (Hz)

EVALUATION _____
_____
_____
_____
_____
_____
_____
_____
_____
_____
_____
_____
_____

INTERPRETATION

RIGHT EAR: Hearing sensitivity is within normal limits with excellent speech discrimination. Middle ear compliance and pressure are normal. The acoustic reflex, however, is absent in this ear.

LEFT EAR: Moderate SN hearing loss in the mid frequencies with mild deficits at 250 Hz and at frequencies above 2000 Hz. The speech discrimination score is good. The results of the Pure Tone Stenger Test (for functional hearing loss) were negative. Middle ear compliance is reduced at slightly negative pressure. The acoustic reflex is absent.

IMPRESSION

Unilateral SN hearing loss following recent head injury.

RECOMMENDATION

Reevaluate hearing status following completion of medical management.

PRESENTING INFORMATION

Pt. and fellow workers suffered with flu-like symptoms for 3 days. On the 3rd day, he called 911 as other employees collapsed. His ears felt full, and he had loud tinnitus, severe headache, and disorientation.

Carbon monoxide poisoning was diagnosed in the ER. He was treated in the hyperbaric oxygen chamber.

Middle ear function is normal, and the acoustic reflex is present without decay AU.

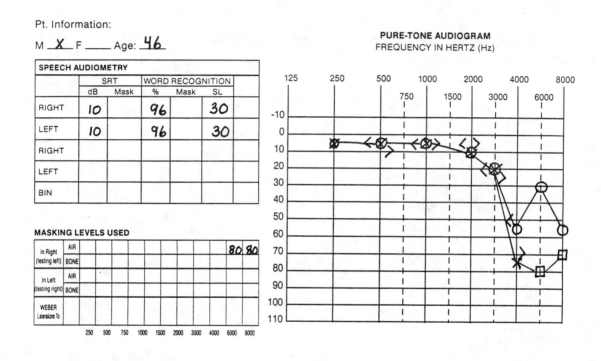

Pt. Information:

M __X__ F _____ Age: __46__

SPEECH AUDIOMETRY

	SRT		WORD RECOGNITION		
	dB	Mask	%	Mask	SL
RIGHT	10		96		30
LEFT	10		96		30
RIGHT					
LEFT					
BIN					

MASKING LEVELS USED

In Right (testing left)	AIR							80	80
	BONE								
In Left (testing right)	AIR								
	BONE								
WEBER Lateralizes To									
		250	500	750	1000	1500	2000	3000	4000	6000	8000

PURE-TONE AUDIOGRAM
FREQUENCY IN HERTZ (Hz)

EVALUATION _____

_____

_____

_____

_____

_____

_____

_____

_____

_____

_____

_____

INTERPRETATION

Test results reveal bilateral normal hearing sensitivity through the low and mid frequencies with mild and moderate high frequency deficits in the right ear and a severe high frequency loss in the left ear. Hearing for speech is normal and speech discrimination scores are very good. Both tympanograms are entirely within normal limits, the acoustic reflex is present through 4000 Hz, AU, and there is no decay of the reflex AU.

OUTCOME

His hearing loss remains stable, and he has explored a variety of treatments for his severe tinnitus.

PRESENTING INFORMATION

This pleasant elderly lady's cc is "swollen glands behind my right ear." Six years ago, a right acoustic neuroma had been diagnosed. She declined treatment. She returned for evaluation one year ago, and, at that time, her right ear test revealed a mild, sloping to severe, SN loss with a 62% discrimination score.

Tympanometry reveals reduced compliance at normal pressure AU. The acoustic reflex is absent AU.

Pt. Information:

M _____ F _X_ Age: _85_

SPEECH AUDIOMETRY

	SRT dB	SRT Mask	WORD RECOGNITION %	WORD RECOGNITION Mask	WORD RECOGNITION SL	
RIGHT	80	75	27	85	25	LOE
LEFT	15		92		30	
RIGHT						
LEFT						
BIN						

MASKING LEVELS USED

In Right (testing left)	AIR									
	BONE									
In Left (testing right)	AIR	75	75		80		90		95	95	95
	BONE		75	→		80				
WEBER Lateralizes To										

250 500 750 1000 1500 2000 3000 4000 6000 8000

PURE-TONE AUDIOGRAM
FREQUENCY IN HERTZ (Hz)

EVALUATION

_____
_____
_____
_____
_____
_____
_____
_____
_____
_____
_____
_____
_____

INTERPRETATION

RIGHT EAR: Severe SN hearing loss with poor speech discrimination. The tympanogram reveals reduced compliance at normal pressure. The acoustic reflex is absent. There had been a 30-35 dB progression in the loss below 1000 Hz, and her speech discrimination ability has dropped significantly.

LEFT EAR: Stable normal hearing thresholds through low and mid frequencies with a precipitous high frequency SN loss. The speech discrimination score is good. Similar to the right ear, the tympanogram reveals reduced compliance at normal pressure, and the acoustic reflex cannot be elicited (in spite of the normal sensitivity through 2000 Hz).

OUTCOME

The radiologist's impression was that the right acoustic neuroma had only a minimal increase in size. The pt. now has a left frontal meningioma. There is also a left pituitary gland lesion (adenoma). She was referred to neurosurgery to discuss treatment options.

PRESENTING INFORMATION

Pt. has a hx of profound hearing loss since birth, secondary to maternal rubella. She currently wears binaural hearing aids and communicates primarily by sign language.

Normal middle ear function AU. No acoustic reflex elicited AU.

Pt. Information:

M ____ F X Age: 40

PURE-TONE AUDIOGRAM
FREQUENCY IN HERTZ (Hz)

SPEECH AUDIOMETRY

	SRT		WORD RECOGNITION			
	dB	Mask	%	Mask	SL	
RIGHT	85		32		20	MCL
LEFT	75		16		25	MCL
RIGHT						
LEFT						
BIN						

MASKING LEVELS USED

In Right (testing left)	AIR										
	BONE										
In Left (testing right)	AIR										
	BONE										
WEBER Lateralizes To											

EVALUATION

INTERPRETATION

Auditory assessment reveals bilateral severe to profound SN hearing loss. Speech discrimination ability is very reduced in the right ear and is poor in the left ear. Acoustic impedance measurements reveal normal middle ear function AU. The acoustic reflex is not elicited AU. This pt. wears well maintained binaural hearing aids. Both earmolds have recently been replaced. Sign language is her preferred method of communication.

She is unemployed and is in the process of obtaining disability determination for SSI benefits.

PRESENTING INFORMATION

Hospital inpatient with 12-day hx of bacterial meningitis and 2-day hx of significant hearing loss. Pt. appeared very ill and uncomfortable (sweating profusely and complaining of severe headache). It was difficult to keep him focused on the test tasks. Same-room testing was necessary. There is no hx of hearing problems prior to this illness.

Normal middle ear function and no acoustic reflex AU.

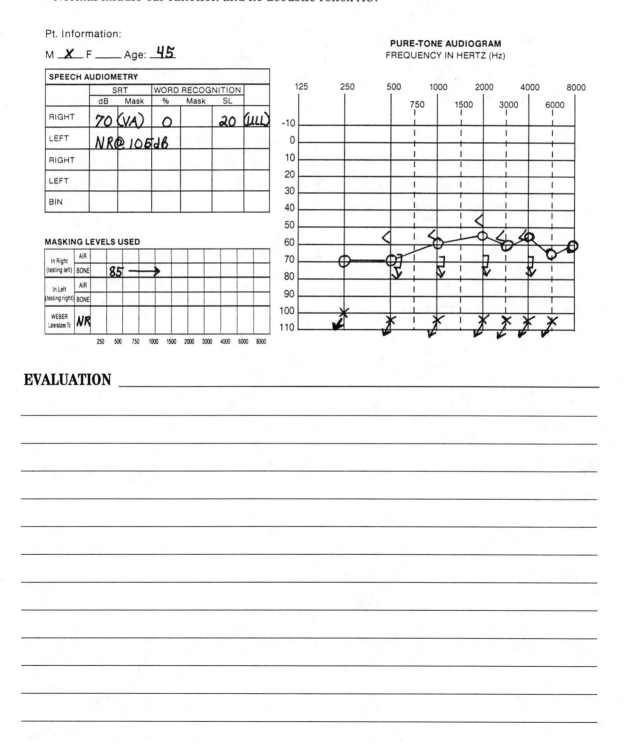

Pt. Information:

M _X_ F _____ Age: _45_

PURE-TONE AUDIOGRAM
FREQUENCY IN HERTZ (Hz)

SPEECH AUDIOMETRY

	SRT		WORD RECOGNITION		
	dB	Mask	%	Mask	SL
RIGHT	70 (VA)		0		20 (ULL)
LEFT	NR@ 105dB				
RIGHT					
LEFT					
BIN					

MASKING LEVELS USED

In Right (testing left)	AIR								
	BONE	85 →							
In Left (testing right)	AIR								
	BONE								
WEBER Lateralizes To	NR								

250 500 750 1000 1500 2000 3000 4000 6000 8000

EVALUATION

INTERPRETATION

RIGHT EAR: Severe SN hearing loss with no speech discrimination ability. Normal middle ear compliance and pressure. There is no acoustic reflex.

LEFT EAR: Profound SN hearing loss. No response to speech testing. Normal middle ear function. No acoustic reflex.

RECOMMENDATIONS

Retest in 48 hours to monitor this severe hearing impairment. He and his family require counseling re his communication and amplification options.

OUTCOME

Subsequent hearing tests revealed similar results. Prior to his transfer to a rehabilitation facility, he was provided with a list and description of assistive listening devices and information about the cochlear implant.

PRESENTING INFORMATION

Progressing unilateral hearing loss, episodes of vertigo with nausea and vomiting, and a sensation of aural fullness. This 27-year-old man is no longer able to work (as an auto mechanic) nor can he trust himself to drive safely.

Normal middle ear function AU. The acoustic reflex is present at each test frequency in each ear and does not decay.

Pt. Information:

M __X__ F _____ Age: **27**

SPEECH AUDIOMETRY

	SRT		WORD RECOGNITION		
	dB	Mask	%	Mask	SL
RIGHT	45	50	76	65	30
LEFT	0		100		30
RIGHT					
LEFT					
BIN					

MASKING LEVELS USED

In Right (testing left) AIR								
In Right (testing left) BONE								
In Left (testing right) AIR	65 →				50 →			
In Left (testing right) BONE		65 →			50			
WEBER Lateralizes To	L							

250 500 750 1000 1500 2000 3000 4000 6000 8000

PURE-TONE AUDIOGRAM
FREQUENCY IN HERTZ (Hz)

EVALUATION

_____

_____

_____

_____

_____

_____

_____

_____

_____

_____

_____

_____

_____

_____

INTERPRETATION

RIGHT EAR: Moderate low- and mid-frequency SN hearing loss which rises to a mild loss above 3000 Hz. The speech discrimination score is fair. Tympanometry reveals normal middle ear pressure and compliance. The acoustic reflex is present and does not decay.

LEFT EAR: Normal hearing sensitivity, excellent speech discrimination score, normal middle ear function and acoustic reflex activity.

IMPRESSION

These test results are consistent with the preliminary diagnosis of Meniere's disease.

OUTCOME

Diagnostic audiologic and radiologic studies supported the diagnosis of Meniere's disease. An endolymphatic shunt surgery was subsequently performed.

PRESENTING INFORMATION

This woman was injured in a MVA 48 hours prior to auditory assessment. Her right cheek and pinna were bruised. She complained of right ear tinnitus and muffled tone quality.

Normal middle ear function but no acoustic reflex AU.

Pt. Information:

M _____ F _X_ Age: _28_

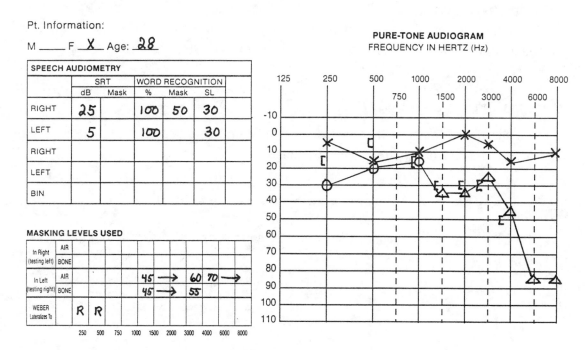

SPEECH AUDIOMETRY

	SRT		WORD RECOGNITION		
	dB	Mask	%	Mask	SL
RIGHT	25		100	50	30
LEFT	5		100		30
RIGHT					
LEFT					
BIN					

MASKING LEVELS USED

In Right (testing left)	AIR							
	BONE							
In Left (testing right)	AIR		·		45 →	60	70 →	
	BONE				45 →	55		
WEBER Lateralizes To	R	R						

250 500 750 1000 1500 2000 3000 4000 6000 8000

EVALUATION

_____

_____

_____

_____

_____

_____

_____

_____

_____

_____

_____

_____

_____

_____

INTERPRETATION

RIGHT EAR: Mild low and mid frequency SN hearing loss with a precipitous drop from moderate to profound impairment at the frequencies above 3000 Hz. The speech discrimination score is excellent. Her middle ear compliance and pressure are within normal limits. There is no acoustic reflex.

LEFT EAR: Normal hearing sensitivity, speech discrimination score, and middle ear compliance and pressure. The ipsilateral acoustic reflex, however, was absent.

IMPRESSIONS

The absence of the acoustic reflex AU is significant. There is a severe unilateral high frequency SN hearing loss following head trauma.

OUTCOME

The CT of the temporal bones was negative: "no temporal bone fx." Pt. did not return for follow-up.

PRESENTING INFORMATION

This 44-year-old woman has advanced ca of the lung with metastasis. She is on the 2nd cycle of chemotherapy. Now complains of tinnitus. No vertigo.

Middle ear function is WNL, AU, and the acoustic reflex is present AU.

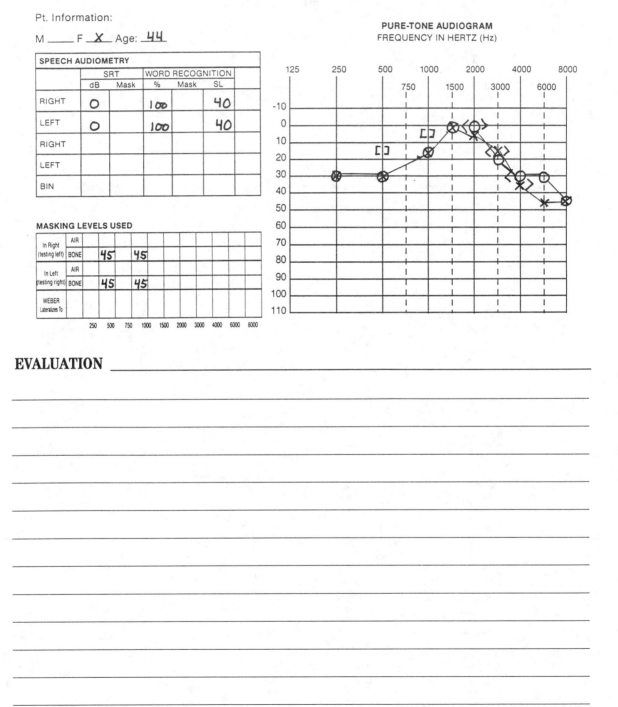

Pt. Information:

M _____ F __X__ Age: __44__

SPEECH AUDIOMETRY

	SRT		WORD RECOGNITION		
	dB	Mask	%	Mask	SL
RIGHT	O		100		40
LEFT	O		100		40
RIGHT					
LEFT					
BIN					

MASKING LEVELS USED

In Right (testing left)	AIR										
	BONE	45		45							
In Left (testing right)	AIR										
	BONE	45		45							
WEBER Lateralizes To											

250 500 750 1000 1500 2000 3000 4000 6000 8000

PURE-TONE AUDIOGRAM
FREQUENCY IN HERTZ (Hz)

EVALUATION _____

_____

_____

_____

_____

_____

_____

_____

_____

_____

_____

_____

_____

_____

_____

INTERPRETATION

Bilateral mild low frequency loss (characterized by a small air-bone gap) and bilateral mild-to-moderate high frequency SN hearing loss. Hearing for speech is within normal limits and speech discrimination scores are excellent. Both tympanograms revealed normal middle ear function and the acoustic reflex is present AU.

RECOMMENDATIONS

Return for monthly monitoring of hearing status. Coping strategies for tinnitus were discussed.

OUTCOME

The pt.'s hx suggests that the hearing loss can be related to her chemotherapy (Cisplatin and UPIG). She did not return for retest. Her prognosis was poor, and it is assumed that she did not survive.

PRESENTING INFORMATION

This 72-year-old woman reports that she has had significant hearing loss for at least 30 years. The onset was gradual. She has a 20-year-old hearing aid for the left ear; the hearing aid is no longer working and cannot be repaired. She is requesting a replacement.

Normal middle ear compliance and pressure AU.

Pt. Information:

M _____ F _X_ Age: _72_

SPEECH AUDIOMETRY

	SRT dB	SRT Mask	WORD RECOGNITION %	WORD RECOGNITION Mask	WORD RECOGNITION SL	
RIGHT	50		52		25	MCL
LEFT	60		52	70	25	↑MCL
RIGHT						
LEFT						
BIN			72		@70 HL	

MASKING LEVELS USED

In Right (testing left)	AIR	75	75							
	BONE		75	→						
In Left (testing right)	AIR									
	BONE									
WEBER Lateralizes To	R									

250 500 750 1000 1500 2000 3000 4000 6000 8000

PURE-TONE AUDIOGRAM
FREQUENCY IN HERTZ (Hz)

EVALUATION

_____

INTERPRETATION

Moderate to severe SN hearing loss in the right ear through the low and mid frequencies; severe SN loss through the low and mid frequencies in the left ear. There is a precipitous drop to a profound impairment at the frequencies above 4000 Hz, bilaterally. Word discrimination scores are severely reduced AU but significantly improve (to "fair") with binaural presentation. Middle ear function is normal AU.

RECOMMENDATIONS

Counseling about and demonstration of binaural hearing aid use.

OUTCOME

This pt. immediately recognized improvement from binaural amplification and updated circuits. She obtained new BTE hearing aids.

PRESENTING INFORMATION

This 39-year-old man was referred by the radiation oncology department. He was scheduled to begin radiation treatment for ca of the right tonsil later the same day. During his pretreatment workup, he reported that he has had a progressing hearing loss.

RIGHT EAR: Normal tympanogram. Acoustic reflex elicited only at 500 Hz with rapid decay.

LEFT EAR: Normal tympanogram and acoustic reflex activity.

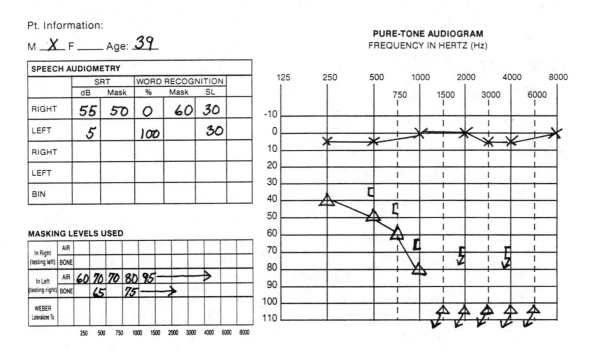

Pt. Information:

M __X__ F _____ Age: **39**

SPEECH AUDIOMETRY

	SRT dB	SRT Mask	WORD RECOGNITION %	WORD RECOGNITION Mask	WORD RECOGNITION SL
RIGHT	55	50	0	60	30
LEFT	5		100		30
RIGHT					
LEFT					
BIN					

MASKING LEVELS USED

		250	500	750	1000	1500	2000	3000	4000	6000	8000
In Right (testing left)	AIR										
	BONE										
In Left (testing right)	AIR	60	70	70	80	95	→				
	BONE		65		75	→					
WEBER Lateralizes To											

PURE-TONE AUDIOGRAM
FREQUENCY IN HERTZ (Hz)

EVALUATION _____

_____

_____

_____

_____

_____

_____

_____

_____

_____

_____

INTERPRETATION

RIGHT EAR: Precipitous, moderate to profound, SN loss with 0% speech discrimination. Middle ear compliance and pressure are normal per tympanometry. The acoustic reflex is elicited only at 500 Hz and shows significant decay.

LEFT EAR: Normal hearing sensitivity, normal hearing for speech, excellent speech discrimination score. Normal middle ear function, normal acoustic reflex thresholds (ipsilateral test). No reflex decay.

IMPRESSION

All right ear test results are consistent with retrocochlear pathology.

RECOMMENDATIONS

Site of lesion evaluation.

OUTCOME

Pt. did not survive.

PRESENTING INFORMATION

This pt. reports having a progressing hearing loss and bilateral constant tinnitus for years. He has a 38-year hx of unprotected exposure to high-level noise in a steel mill.

Normal middle ear function AU. The acoustic reflex is elicited, without decay, through 2K Hz, AD, and through 1K Hz, AS.

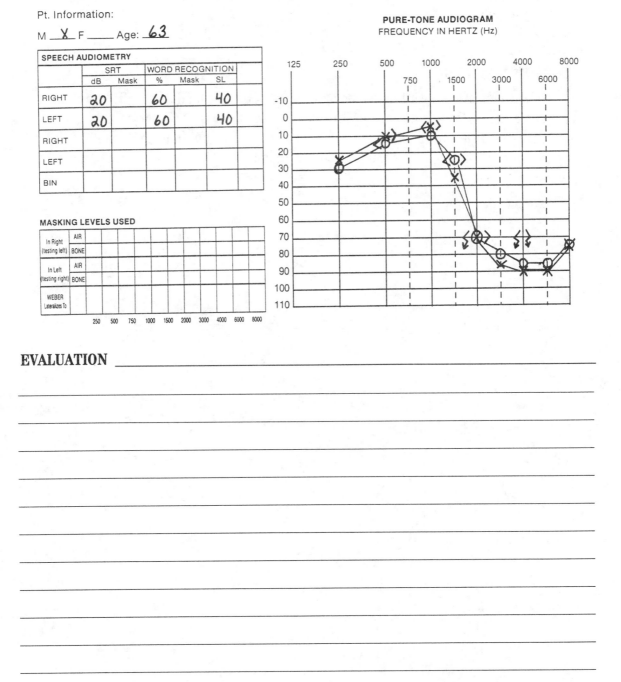

Pt. Information:

M __X__ F ____ Age: __63__

SPEECH AUDIOMETRY

	SRT		WORD RECOGNITION		
	dB	Mask	%	Mask	SL
RIGHT	20		60		40
LEFT	20		60		40
RIGHT					
LEFT					
BIN					

MASKING LEVELS USED

In Right (testing left)	AIR								
	BONE								
In Left (testing right)	AIR								
	BONE								
WEBER Lateralizes To									
	250	500	750	1000	1500	2000	3000	4000	6000 8000

PURE-TONE AUDIOGRAM
FREQUENCY IN HERTZ (Hz)

EVALUATION

INTERPRETATION

Auditory assessment reveals normal hearing sensitivity only at 500 and 1000 Hz. There is a mild deficit at 250 Hz and a precipitous, mild to profound, sensori-neural loss above 1000 Hz. The speech discrimination scores are significantly reduced AU. Tympanometry reveals normal middle ear compliance and pressure for both ears. The acoustic reflex is present through 2000 Hz in the right ear and through 1000 Hz in the left ear. There is no decay of the reflex AU.

RECOMMENDATIONS

He was counseled regarding the need for hearing protection devices (HPD's) in high-level noise areas. He was given literature about hearing loss and hearing aids and was advised to arrange an appointment for a hearing aid evaluation. It is possible that amplification will help mask his tinnitus along with improving his ability to communicate.

PRESENTING INFORMATION

Child with congenital hearing loss and deformed pinnas. She has one hearing aid. There are no known special services provided at school (no FM system, no tutoring, no speech therapy).

Normal tympanograms. The acoustic reflex is present at 500 and 1K Hz, AU.

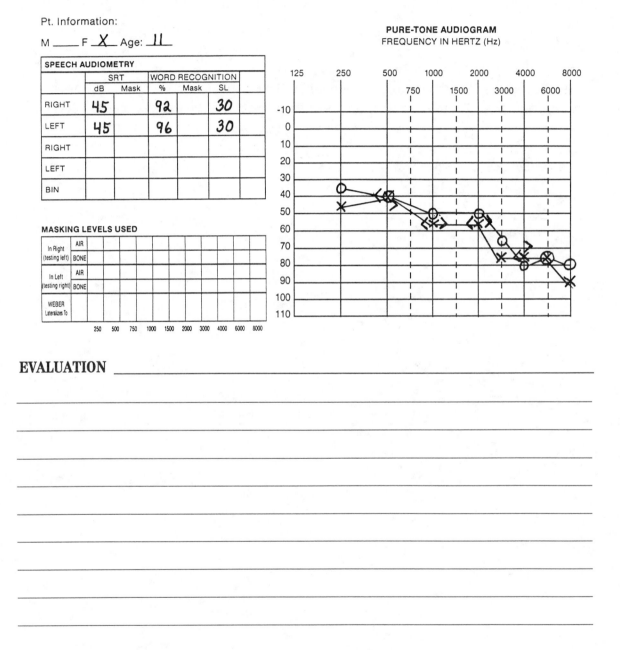

Pt. Information:

M _____ F _X_ Age: _11_

SPEECH AUDIOMETRY

	SRT		WORD RECOGNITION		
	dB	Mask	%	Mask	SL
RIGHT	45		92		30
LEFT	45		96		30
RIGHT					
LEFT					
BIN					

MASKING LEVELS USED

In Right (testing left)	AIR									
	BONE									
In Left (testing right)	AIR									
	BONE									
WEBER Lateralizes To										
		250	500	750	1000	1500	2000	3000	4000	6000	8000

PURE-TONE AUDIOGRAM
FREQUENCY IN HERTZ (Hz)

EVALUATION

_____

_____

_____

_____

_____

_____

_____

_____

_____

_____

_____

_____

_____

_____

INTERPRETATION

The auditory assessment reveals bilateral mild, sloping to severe-profound, SN hearing loss. There is a moderate to severe loss in the speech frequencies with good word discrimination ability. The tympanogram for each ear reveals normal middle ear compliance and pressure. The acoustic reflex is present at 500 and 1000 Hz (only)AU.

RECOMMENDATIONS

Evaluate performance with present hearing aid. Obtain funding for binaural amplification. Mother advised to apply for SSI for the child. Information re the education of hearing handicapped children was sent via the mother to the school. The school principal was contacted re this child's need for special seating and consideration in the classroom and for special services and equipment.

PRESENTING INFORMATION

This is the 3rd audiologic evaluation within 6 months for this woman who has noticed a progressing right ear hearing loss since the birth of her baby 11 months ago. The previous audiograms identified a sloping right SN loss with excellent, then later, fair, speech discrimination score, and abnormal acoustic reflex activity. Normal middle ear function AU. The left ipsilateral acoustic reflex does not decay; right ipsilateral reflexes decay rapidly.

Pt. Information:

M _____ F _X_ Age: _29_

SPEECH AUDIOMETRY

	SRT dB	SRT Mask	WORD RECOGNITION %	WORD RECOGNITION Mask	WORD RECOGNITION SL
RIGHT	45	40	44	60	30
LEFT	10		96		30
RIGHT					
LEFT					
BIN					

MASKING LEVELS USED

		250	500	750	1000	1500	2000	3000	4000	6000	8000
In Right (testing left)	AIR										
	BONE										
In Left (testing right)	AIR	65	60		50		60	60	65	→	70
	BONE		60/65	→							
WEBER Lateralizes To											

PURE-TONE AUDIOGRAM
FREQUENCY IN HERTZ (Hz)

EVALUATION

_____

_____

_____

_____

_____

_____

_____

_____

_____

_____

_____

INTERPRETATION

RIGHT EAR: There has been further significant progression in the hearing loss. There is now a flat, moderately-severe SN loss. There has been a further decline (from 56% to 44%) in word discrimination. The tympanogram is normal. The acoustic reflex rapidly decays with tone right.

LEFT EAR: All test results remain within normal limits. The acoustic reflex is present, tone left, and does not decay.

OUTCOME

The MRI revealed no pathology. The VDRL was nonreactive. No diagnosis has been made at this time. She has been loaned a hearing aid for the right ear (to mask her severe tinnitus and to assist her directional hearing).

PRESENTING INFORMATION

Pt. is an insulin-dependent diabetic with progressing hearing loss. In addition to his hearing loss, he is experiencing increasing problems with his vision.

Both tympanograms are WNL. The acoustic reflex is present through 2K Hz AU and does not decay.

Pt. Information:

M _X_ F ____ Age: _72_

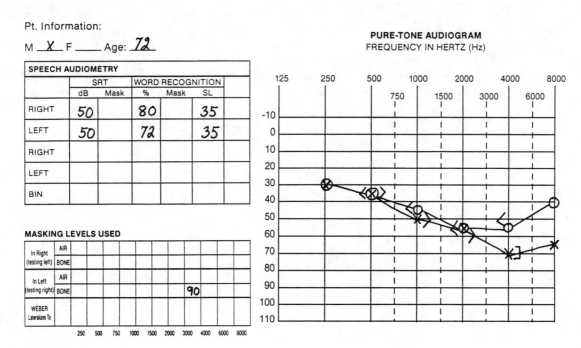

SPEECH AUDIOMETRY

	SRT		WORD RECOGNITION			
	dB	Mask	%	Mask	SL	
RIGHT	50		80		35	
LEFT	50		72		35	
RIGHT						
LEFT						
BIN						

MASKING LEVELS USED

In Right (testing left)	AIR									
	BONE									
In Left (testing right)	AIR									
	BONE					90				
WEBER Lateralizes To										
		250	500	750	1000	1500	2000	3000	4000	6000	8000

PURE-TONE AUDIOGRAM
FREQUENCY IN HERTZ (Hz)

EVALUATION

_____

_____

_____

_____

_____

_____

_____

_____

_____

_____

_____

_____

INTERPRETATION

RIGHT EAR: Mild-to-moderate SN hearing loss with fairly good speech discrimination.

LEFT EAR: Mild-to-severe SN hearing loss with fair speech discrimination. Middle ear measures are normal AU. The acoustic reflex is present through 2000 Hz AU and does not decay.

RECOMMENDATIONS

Amplification for the right ear (with medical clearance). The pt. has Medicaid, which will provide one hearing aid.

PRESENTING INFORMATION

Multiple gunshot wounds to right side of face 8-9 years ago. Blinded in right eye. One bullet on a downward projectory through the right eye remains. Location of bullet unknown (records at out-of-state site). He reports that right ear hearing was immediately affected. There has been progression in bilateral hearing loss accompanied by frontal headaches and tinnitus.

The tympanograms are WNL, and the acoustic reflex is absent AU.

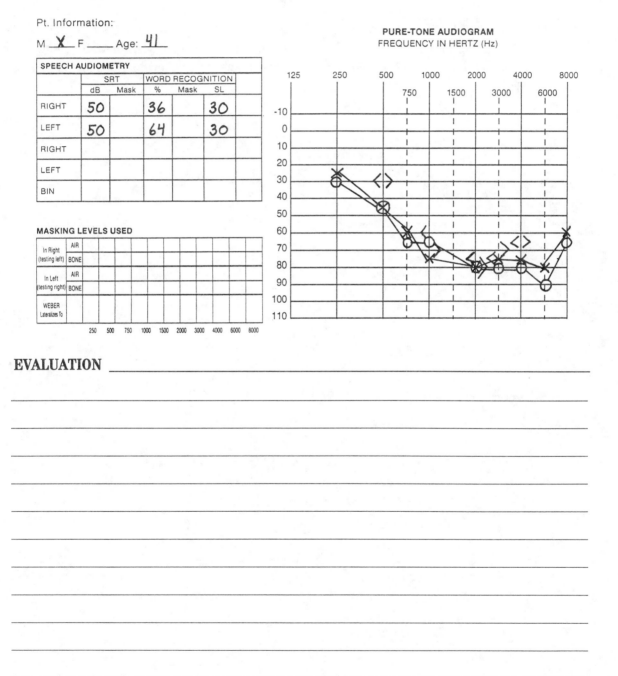

Pt. Information:

M __X__ F _____ Age: __41__

SPEECH AUDIOMETRY

	SRT		WORD RECOGNITION		
	dB	Mask	%	Mask	SL
RIGHT	50		36		30
LEFT	50		64		30
RIGHT					
LEFT					
BIN					

MASKING LEVELS USED

In Right (testing left)	AIR										
	BONE										
In Left (testing right)	AIR										
	BONE										
WEBER Lateralizes To											

250 500 750 1000 1500 2000 3000 4000 6000 8000

PURE-TONE AUDIOGRAM
FREQUENCY IN HERTZ (Hz)

EVALUATION

INTERPRETATION

There is a bilateral mild-to-moderate low frequency deficit falling to a moderately-severe, or severe, SN loss through the mid and high frequencies. Hearing for speech is moderately impaired; speech discrimination is poor in the right ear and significantly reduced in the left. Middle ear measures are within normal limits AU.

The acoustic reflex is absent AU.

IMPRESSION/ RECOMMENDATION

Severe hearing impairment. Asymmetrical poor/reduced word discrimination. Needs referral for binaural hearing aids when the site of lesion and medical evaluations have been completed.

PRESENTING INFORMATION

Pt. reports a "lifetime" of asymmetrical hearing loss. His better (left) ear has been fit with hearing aids for the past 20 years. Recently, he has noticed the onset of constant tinnitus and a progression in the hearing loss in each ear. He is HIV positive.

Normal tympanograms. The acoustic reflex is present AU.

Pt. Information:

M _X_ F _____ Age: _41_

SPEECH AUDIOMETRY

	SRT		WORD RECOGNITION		
	dB	Mask	%	Mask	SL
RIGHT	50	50	80	65	30
LEFT	25		92		30
RIGHT					
LEFT					
BIN					

MASKING LEVELS USED

		250	500	750	1000	1500	2000	3000	4000	6000	8000
In Right (testing left)	AIR										
	BONE										
In Left (testing right)	AIR	65	65		65		70/75	80 →			
	BONE		75	→				85			
WEBER Lateralizes To		L	✓		✓						

PURE-TONE AUDIOGRAM
FREQUENCY IN HERTZ (Hz)

EVALUATION

_____

_____

_____

_____

_____

_____

_____

_____

_____

_____

_____

_____

_____

INTERPRETATION

RIGHT EAR: Moderate-severe SN hearing loss with fair speech discrimination.

LEFT EAR: Mild to moderately-severe SN loss with good speech discrimination Both ears have normal middle ear measurements. The acoustic reflex is elicited at 500 and 1000 Hz AU. There was some debris (suspect fungus) in the right ear canal (which may account for the small low frequency air-bone gap in that ear).

RECOMMENDATION

ENT consult regarding asymmetrical hearing loss-progressing. Return to audiology for assessment of amplification needs.

PRESENTING INFORMATION

This teenager presents with the cc of bilateral, constant, moderately-severe tinnitus. He has (mild) cerebral palsy and a seizure disorder. He states that the tinnitus impairs his concentration and causes delayed and disturbed sleep.

Tympanograms are WNL, and acoustic reflexes are elicited AU.

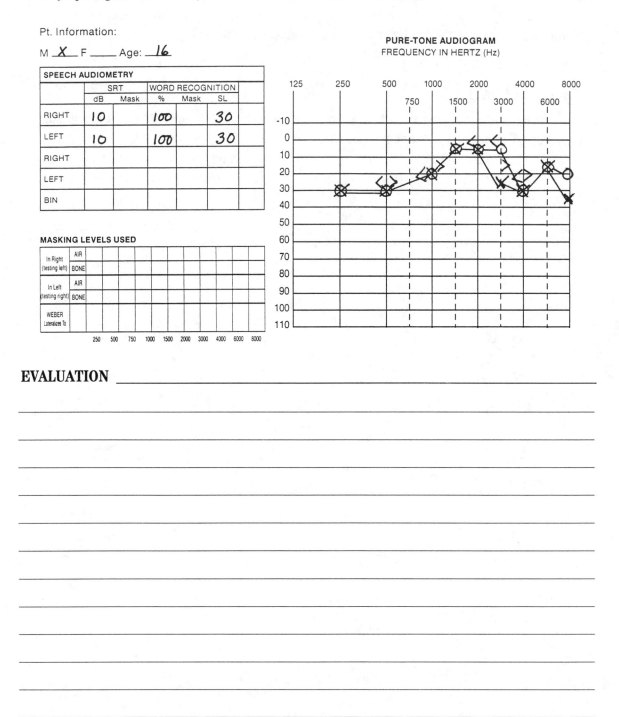

Pt. Information:

M _X_ F ____ Age: _16_

SPEECH AUDIOMETRY

	SRT		WORD RECOGNITION		
	dB	Mask	%	Mask	SL
RIGHT	10		100		30
LEFT	10		100		30
RIGHT					
LEFT					
BIN					

MASKING LEVELS USED

In Right (testing left)	AIR									
	BONE									
In Left (testing right)	AIR									
	BONE									
WEBER Lateralizes To										
		250	500	750	1000	1500	2000	3000	4000	6000	8000

PURE-TONE AUDIOGRAM
FREQUENCY IN HERTZ (Hz)

EVALUATION _____

_____

_____

_____

_____

_____

_____

_____

_____

_____

_____

_____

_____

INTERPRETATION

Auditory assessment reveals bilateral mild SN hearing loss with the exception of some normal sensitivity in the mid frequencies. His speech reception thresholds reflect his efficient use of these mid-frequency cues. His speech discrimination scores are excellent. Tympanometry reveals normal middle ear function. Acoustic reflexes are elicited AU. His tinnitus is matched at 12,000 Hz and cannot be effectively masked.

RECOMMENDATIONS

He has been referred back to the physician who evaluates and manages his seizure disorder to check his current medications for tinnitus as a side effect. Although it is believed that he has always had some slight hearing impairment, it has never been routinely monitored. Annual hearing tests are recommended. Tinnitus coping strategies were discussed.

PRESENTING INFORMATION

This young woman awoke (6 hours before this test) with hissing tinnitus and sudden right ear hearing loss. There is no hx of aural pain, trauma, or infection.

Normal tympanograms. The acoustic reflex is present in the left ear and is absent in the right ear.

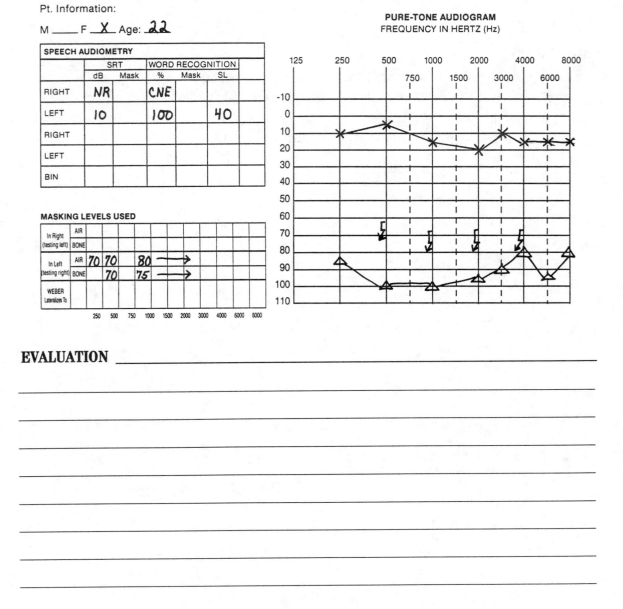

Pt. Information:

M _____ F _X_ Age: _22_

SPEECH AUDIOMETRY

	SRT dB	SRT Mask	WORD RECOGNITION %	WORD RECOGNITION Mask	SL
RIGHT	NR		CNE		
LEFT	10		100		40
RIGHT					
LEFT					
BIN					

MASKING LEVELS USED

In Right (testing left) AIR										
In Right (testing left) BONE										
In Left (testing right) AIR	70	70		80	→					
In Left (testing right) BONE		70		75	→					
WEBER Lateralizes To										

250 500 750 1000 1500 2000 3000 4000 6000 8000

PURE-TONE AUDIOGRAM
FREQUENCY IN HERTZ (Hz)

EVALUATION

_____

_____

_____

_____

_____

_____

_____

_____

_____

_____

_____

_____

INTERPRETATION

The auditory assessment reveals a normal audiogram and excellent word discrimination for the left ear. The right ear results indicate a profound SN loss of hearing with no speech discrimination ability. Both ears have normal middle ear compliance and pressure. The acoustic reflex is present in the left ear and is absent in the right ear (consistent with the severity of the right ear hearing loss).

OUTCOME

This sudden loss was treated with steroids and responded well. The pt. realized improvement to a mild loss in the left ear within one month.

PRESENTING INFORMATION

This pt. complains of severe pain in each ear and aural fullness.
Both tympanograms reflect normal middle ear function.

Pt. Information:

M _____ F _X_ Age: _40_

PURE-TONE AUDIOGRAM
FREQUENCY IN HERTZ (Hz)

SPEECH AUDIOMETRY

	SRT		WORD RECOGNITION		
	dB	Mask	%	Mask	SL
RIGHT	10		100		30
LEFT	10		100		30
RIGHT					
LEFT					
BIN					

MASKING LEVELS USED

In Right (testing left)	AIR									
	BONE									
In Left (testing right)	AIR									
	BONE									
WEBER Lateralizes To										

250   500   750   1000   1500   2000   3000   4000   6000   8000

EVALUATION

INTERPRETATION

Test results reveal bilateral normal hearing sensitivity through 4000 Hz with a mild-moderate high frequency SN deficit. Hearing for speech is within normal limits, and speech discrimination scores are excellent. The tympanograms were essentially WNL.

OUTCOME

The physical examination revealed that the patient has severe tympromandibular joint dysfunction (TMJ). She was referred to oral surgery for evaluation.

PRESENTING INFORMATION

"Years" of bilateral tinnitus which seems to be increasing in annoyance. Since menopause, she has had difficulty with waking several times a night. The tinnitus causes her to have trouble falling asleep again. She seeks evaluation and management of this problem. Her hearing status has been evaluated in the past, and she has been told that she had a slight loss.

Middle ear compliance and pressure are WNL AU.

Pt. Information:

M _____ F _X_ Age: _57_

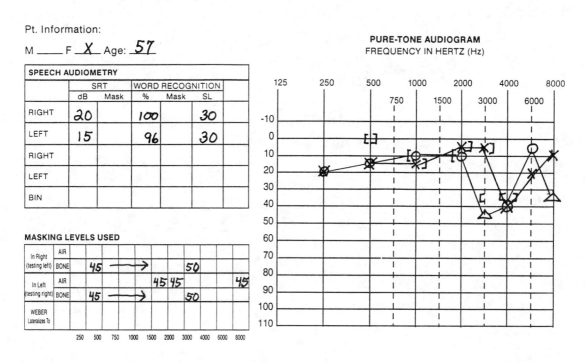

SPEECH AUDIOMETRY

	SRT		WORD RECOGNITION		
	dB	Mask	%	Mask	SL
RIGHT	20		100		30
LEFT	15		96		30
RIGHT					
LEFT					
BIN					

MASKING LEVELS USED

In Right (testing left)	AIR								
	BONE	45 →				50			
In Left (testing right)	AIR				45	45			45
	BONE	45 →				50			
WEBER Lateralizes To									

250 500 750 1000 1500 2000 3000 4000 6000 8000

EVALUATION _____

_____

_____

_____

_____

_____

_____

_____

_____

_____

_____

_____

INTERPRETATION

The auditory assessment reveals a mild-moderate high frequency SN deficit in each ear. Through the low and mid frequencies, hearing sensitivity is WNL. Hearing for speech is very mildly impaired. Speech discrimination scores are very good. Tympanometry reveals normal middle ear pressure and compliance AU.

IMPRESSION

Peculiar pattern of high frequency SN hearing loss.

OUTCOME

A detailed medical hx revealed that she had several years of occult CO poisoning (faulty furnace) at the time the tinnitus and hearing difficulties were noticed. Her diagnostic tests have negative findings for retrocochlear pathology. The CO poisoning is considered to be of possible significance in her case. Tinnitus management has been inititiated.

PRESENTING INFORMATION

This lady had been evaluated in the ENT Clinic several years ago. She subsequently obtained a hearing aid and did not return for follow up. Now, over 4 years later, she has lost the aid and seeks replacement.

Tympanograms are normal. There is no acoustic reflex above 1K Hz, AD, or above 500 Hz, AS.

Pt. Information:

M _____ F _X_ Age: _61_

SPEECH AUDIOMETRY

	SRT		WORD RECOGNITION		
	dB	Mask	%	Mask	SL
RIGHT	25		88		30
LEFT	30		76		30
RIGHT					
LEFT			64	70	35
BIN					

MASKING LEVELS USED

In Right (testing left)	AIR	50				55	70	85	→
	BONE		55		55	65		75	
In Left (testing right)	AIR								
	BONE								
WEBER Lateralizes To									

250 500 750 1000 1500 2000 3000 4000 6000 8000

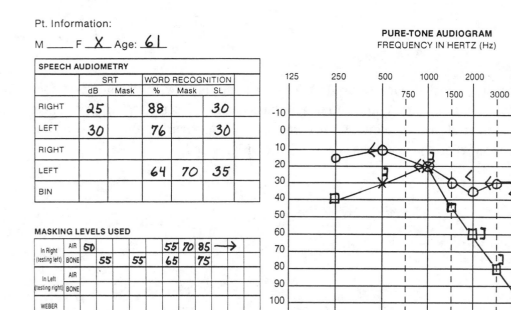

PURE-TONE AUDIOGRAM
FREQUENCY IN HERTZ (Hz)

EVALUATION _____

INTERPRETATION

RIGHT EAR: Mild SN hearing loss at frequencies above 1K Hz. Fairly good speech discrimination. Normal tympanogram. No acoustic reflex above 1K Hz.

LEFT EAR: Mild low frequency SN loss with a precipitous drop to a profound, high frequency SN loss. Speech discrimination ability is only fair and deteriorates at a higher presentation level (PI-PB rollover). The tympanogram is normal. There is no acoustic reflex above 500 Hz.

IMPRESSION

The asymmetrical, progressing left ear hearing loss with reduced speech discrimination, positive rollover, and absence of the acoustic reflex suggests retrocochlear site of lesion. Special tests of auditory function are indicated. Hearing aid evaluation and recommendation is postponed until medical clearance is provided.

PRESENTING INFORMATION

This is this pt.'s 3rd hearing evaluation in 5 years. A teacher, he complains of difficulty hearing students, and he cleverly manipulates classroom seating and social situations to avoid difficult listening situations. He has been unable to accept his need for amplification. He has a significant hx of service-related noise exposure. He denies a family hx of hearing loss.

Normal middle ear compliance and pressure AU. The acoustic reflex is elicited AU.

Pt. Information:

M _X_ F ____ Age: __68__

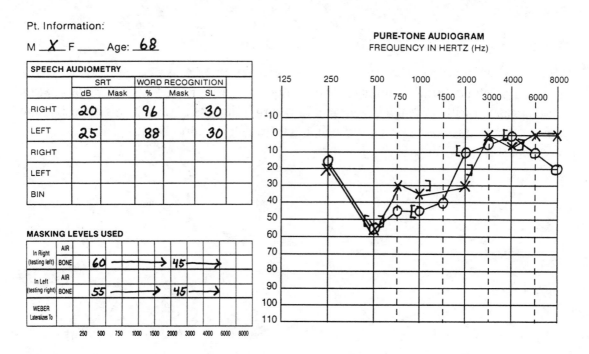

SPEECH AUDIOMETRY					
	SRT		WORD RECOGNITION		
	dB	Mask	%	Mask	SL
RIGHT	20		96		30
LEFT	25		88		30
RIGHT					
LEFT					
BIN					

MASKING LEVELS USED

In Right (testing left)	AIR							
	BONE	60 ——————→		45 ——————→				
In Left (testing right)	AIR							
	BONE	55 ——————→		45 ——————→				
WEBER Lateralizes To								

250 500 750 1000 1500 2000 3000 4000 6000 8000

EVALUATION
_____

_____

_____

_____

_____

_____

_____

_____

_____

_____

INTERPRETATION

Auditory assessment reveals bilateral moderate to mild SN hearing loss in the mid frequencies (only). Hearing for speech is mildly impaired. The right ear speech discrimination score is very good; the left ear score is fairly good. Tympanometry reveals normal middle ear function AU. The acoustic reflex is elicited AU. The etiology of this loss has never been established. The slight, but persistent, asymmetry in speech discrimination ability, together with the unusual contour of the loss, suggests the need for site of lesion evaluation.

OUTCOME

The pt. did return for a demonstration and discussion of his various amplification options but left without making a decision. He stated that his physician was going to refer him to an otologist for evaluation but had a "low level of concern" because the hearing loss has remained stable for years.

PRESENTING INFORMATION

Pt. wears a right ear hearing aid. She is referred for hearing evaluation and medical clearance necessary for replacement of the aid "which don't do me no good."

Both tympanograms are normal. The acoustic reflex is present at elevated threshold levels AU.

Pt. Information:

M _____ F _X_ Age: _57_

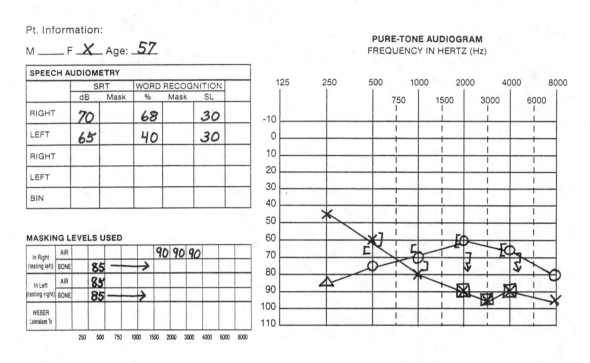

SPEECH AUDIOMETRY

	SRT		WORD RECOGNITION		
	dB	Mask	%	Mask	SL
RIGHT	70		68		30
LEFT	65		40		30
RIGHT					
LEFT					
BIN					

MASKING LEVELS USED

						90	90	90				
In Right (testing left)	AIR					90	90	90				
	BONE	85 →										
In Left (testing right)	AIR	85										
	BONE	85 →										
WEBER Lateralizes To												

250 500 750 1000 1500 2000 3000 4000 6000 8000

PURE-TONE AUDIOGRAM
FREQUENCY IN HERTZ (Hz)

EVALUATION

_____

_____

_____

_____

_____

_____

_____

_____

_____

_____

_____

_____

_____

INTERPRETATION

Bilateral severe SN hearing loss with reduced speech discrimination ability, right ear, and a poor discrimination score, left ear. Middle ear compliance and pressure are WNL AU. The acoustic reflex is present (at elevated levels) AU.

OUTCOME

Positive VDRL. The hearing loss is attributed to otosyphillis. Hearing status will be monitored during treatment.

PRESENTING INFORMATION

Hx of bilateral otosclerosis and bilateral stapedectomy. Pt. has developed severe vertigo. He is unable to drive because of this. The ENG reveals significant right ear weakness. He has been wearing powerful BTE hearing aids for one year.

Both tympanograms reflect normal middle ear compliance and pressure.

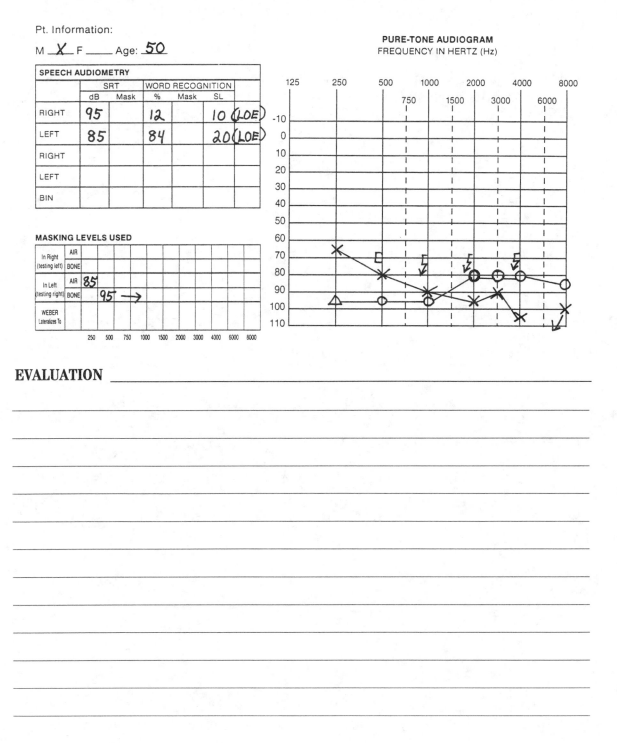

Pt. Information:

M __X__ F _____ Age: __50__

SPEECH AUDIOMETRY

	SRT		WORD RECOGNITION		
	dB	Mask	%	Mask	SL
RIGHT	95		12		10 (LOE)
LEFT	85		84		20 (LOE)
RIGHT					
LEFT					
BIN					

MASKING LEVELS USED

In Right (testing left)	AIR										
	BONE										
In Left (testing right)	AIR	85									
	BONE		95 →								
WEBER Lateralizes To											
		250	500	750	1000	1500	2000	3000	4000	6000	8000

EVALUATION
_____

_____

_____

_____

_____

_____

_____

_____

_____

_____

_____

_____

_____

INTERPRETATION

Auditory assessment reveals bilateral severe-profound SN hearing loss. He has very poor speech discrimination in the right ear and good discrimination, left ear. Both tympanograms reflect normal middle ear pressure and compliance. Fistula tests were negative AU.

OUTCOME

Pt. declined the recommended labyrinthectomy. He was placed on Valium which is keeping the vertigo in check. "He is able to function."

PRESENTING INFORMATION

Pt. referred by a nursing home with the following diagnoses: bronchitis, manic-depressive psychosis, s/p right cerebral thombosis, Parkinson's disease, hearing loss, and cataracts.

Pt. Information:

M _____ F __X__ Age: __71__

SPEECH AUDIOMETRY

	SRT		WORD RECOGNITION			
	dB	Mask	%	Mask	SL	
RIGHT	95	(VA)	NR		10	LOE
LEFT	90	(VA)	NR		15	LOE
RIGHT						
LEFT						
BIN						

MASKING LEVELS USED

In Right (testing left)	AIR									
	BONE									
In Left (testing right)	AIR									
	BONE									
WEBER Lateralizes To										
		250	500	750	1000	1500	2000	3000	4000	6000	8000

PURE-TONE AUDIOGRAM
FREQUENCY IN HERTZ (Hz)

EVALUATION

INTERPRETATION

This pt. required modified test techniques and instructions. These results are of only fair reliability. (She cannot understand the tasks involved in these tests.) The test results suggest that she has bilateral severe-to-profound SN hearing loss. There was no response to bone conduction testing. She demonstrated voice awareness but appears to have no speech discrimination ability.

OUTCOME

We learned that this pt. has a hearing aid in good condition and that the nursing home has also tried an amplifier with a headset on her. She will not wear either device. Her nurse has observed no change in auditory awareness with amplification.

PRESENTING INFORMATION

Trauma to face and head two days ago. There are multiple facial fractures including a depressed fx of the left zygomatic arch. Pt. was very uncomfortable, and his eyes were swollen shut. He was alert and cooperative.

Normal right tympanogram. He could not tolerate the probe in the left canal.

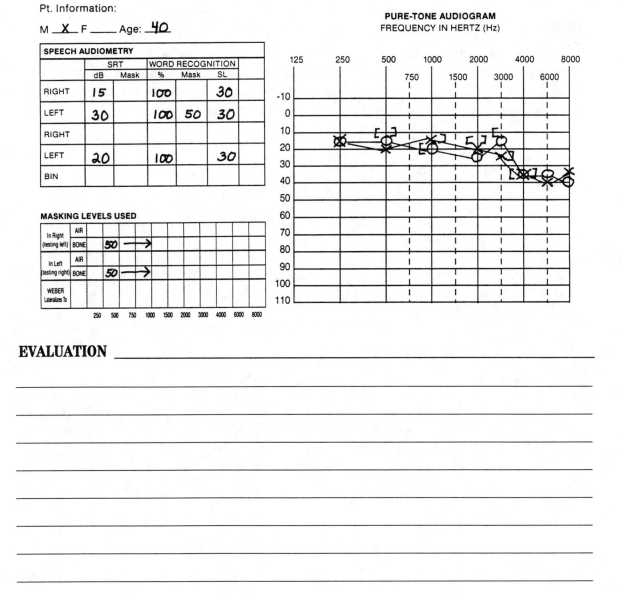

Pt. Information:

M __X__ F _____ Age: __40__

SPEECH AUDIOMETRY

	SRT		WORD RECOGNITION		
	dB	Mask	%	Mask	SL
RIGHT	15		100		30
LEFT	30		100	50	30
RIGHT					
LEFT	20		100		30
BIN					

MASKING LEVELS USED

In Right (testing left)	AIR								
	BONE	50 →							
In Left (testing right)	AIR								
	BONE	50 →							
WEBER Lateralizes To									

250 500 750 1000 1500 2000 3000 4000 6000 8000

PURE-TONE AUDIOGRAM
FREQUENCY IN HERTZ (Hz)

EVALUATION _____

_____

_____

_____

_____

_____

_____

_____

_____

_____

_____

_____

_____

INTERPRETATION

Hearing sensitivity is WNL through 3000 Hz AU. There is a mild high-frequency SN deficit, bilaterally. Hearing for speech is at normal limits; speech discrimination scores are excellent. The right tympanogram is normal. We could not assess the left ear's status as he could not tolerate the probe.

OUTCOME

He returned to clinic several times for management of his facial injuries. He had no further complaints about his ear or his hearing status.

PRESENTING INFORMATION

Hearing evaluation prior to selection of binaural hearing aids. Speech quality and articulation errors are consistent with congenital hearing loss. He has dropped out of high school.

Middle ear function is WNL AU. The acoustic reflex is not elicited AU.

Pt. Information:

M _X_ F _____ Age: _17_

PURE-TONE AUDIOGRAM
FREQUENCY IN HERTZ (Hz)

SPEECH AUDIOMETRY

	SRT		WORD RECOGNITION		
	dB	Mask	%	Mask	SL
RIGHT	45		42		30
LEFT	50		40		30
RIGHT					
LEFT					
BIN					

MASKING LEVELS USED

In Right (testing left)	AIR								
	BONE								
In Left (testing right)	AIR								
	BONE								
WEBER Lateralizes To									
		250	500	750	1000	1500	2000	3000	4000	6000	8000

EVALUATION _____

_____

_____

_____

_____

_____

_____

_____

_____

_____

_____

_____

_____

_____

INTERPRETATION

Test results reveal bilateral moderate-to-severe SN hearing loss. Speech discrimination scores are significantly reduced AU. Middle ear compliance and pressure are WNL AU. The acoustic reflex is not elicited AU.

OUTCOME

The family hx reveals a paternal familial loss which is present in 4 living relatives and which presents as a severe impairment in each case. This pt. was provided with information regarding genetic counseling opportunities. His current audiometric results were explained. Referral to the BVR was completed. Binaural hearing aids were requested.

PRESENTING INFORMATION

Pt. reports having suffered a CVA 5 years ago with residual right facial weakness and incomplete eye closure. His chief complaints concern the onset of gait instability and a loud right ear tinnitus, which began 8 months ago.

Middle ear compliance and pressure are WNL AU. The acoustic reflex is absent in each ear with ipsilateral and contralateral presentations.

Pt. Information:

M _X_ F _____ Age: **60**

SPEECH AUDIOMETRY

	SRT dB	SRT Mask	WORD RECOGNITION %	WORD RECOGNITION Mask	SL
RIGHT	10		100		30
LEFT	15		92		30
RIGHT			96	55	60
LEFT			96	55	60
BIN					

MASKING LEVELS USED

In Right (testing left)	AIR									
	BONE									
In Left (testing right)	AIR		·							
	BONE									
WEBER Lateralizes To										
		250	500	750	1000	1500	2000	3000	4000	6000	8000

PURE-TONE AUDIOGRAM
FREQUENCY IN HERTZ (Hz)

EVALUATION

INTERPRETATION

Auditory assessment reveals bilateral essentially normal hearing thresholds through the low and mid frequencies with a moderate-severe SN deficit at the frequencies above 3000 Hz. His speech discrimination scores are very good, and a check for PI-PB rollover is negative. Both tympanograms are WNL. The acoustic reflex is absent AU. These test results are stable compared to his evaluation 3 years ago.

OUTCOME

Large right CPA tumor displacing pons. Referred to neurosurgery for evaluation.

PRESENTING INFORMATION

S/P gunshot wound to left tragus. Bullet under skin of left cheek. Bullet was surgically removed 4 days ago. Entrance wounds healing well. Testing of the left ear was accomplished with a cushioned headset and hand supported earphone (with a sterile cover) to protect his painful ear and cheek.

The right tympanogram was normal. CNT left ear.

Pt. Information:

M __X__ F ____ Age: __37__

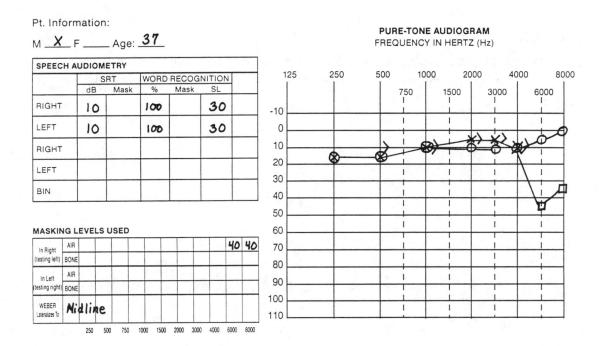

SPEECH AUDIOMETRY

	SRT		WORD RECOGNITION		
	dB	Mask	%	Mask	SL
RIGHT	10		100		30
LEFT	10		100		30
RIGHT					
LEFT					
BIN					

MASKING LEVELS USED

In Right (testing left)	AIR							40	40
	BONE								
In Left (testing right)	AIR								
	BONE								
WEBER Lateralizes To	Midline								

250 500 750 1000 1500 2000 3000 4000 6000 8000

PURE-TONE AUDIOGRAM
FREQUENCY IN HERTZ (Hz)

EVALUATION _____

_____

_____

_____

_____

_____

_____

_____

_____

_____

_____

INTERPRETATION

Auditory assessment reveals normal hearing sensitivity, speech discrimination ability, and middle ear function for the right ear. Left ear hearing sensitivity is WNL except for a mild-moderate deficit above 4000 Hz. Speech discrimination is not affected. Tympanometry was not attempted due to the condition of the tragus.

OUTCOME

The pt.'s wounds healed quickly. A repeated hearing test continued to reveal a high-frequency deficit in the left ear. It is possible that it is due to noise trauma from the gunshot.

PRESENTING INFORMATION

Sudden (paroxysmal) drop in left ear hearing sensitivity following deep sea diving. She was also experiencing dizziness and unstable gait.

Normal right and left middle ear function. Positive fistula test, left ear.

Pt. Information:

M _____ F __X__ Age: __30__

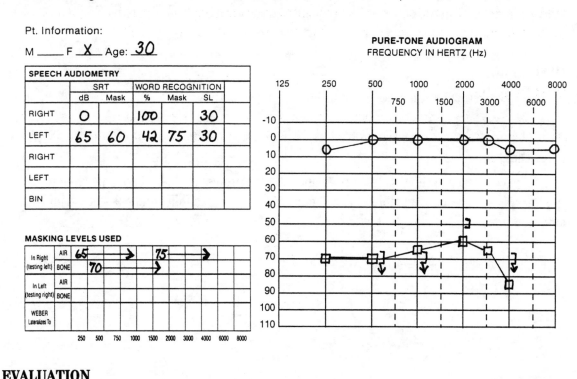

SPEECH AUDIOMETRY

	SRT		WORD RECOGNITION		
	dB	Mask	%	Mask	SL
RIGHT	O		100		30
LEFT	65	60	42	75	30
RIGHT					
LEFT					
BIN					

MASKING LEVELS USED

		250	500	750	1000	1500	2000	3000	4000	6000	8000
In Right (testing left)	AIR	65 →→			75 →→						
	BONE	70 →→									
In Left (testing right)	AIR										
	BONE										
WEBER Lateralizes To											

PURE-TONE AUDIOGRAM
FREQUENCY IN HERTZ (Hz)

EVALUATION _____

_____
_____
_____
_____
_____
_____
_____
_____
_____
_____
_____
_____
_____

INTERPRETATION

RIGHT EAR: Normal audiogram, word discrimination and middle ear function.

LEFT EAR: Severe SN hearing loss 250 through 4000 Hz with a profound deficit at higher frequencies. Word discrimination ability is poor. The acoustic impedance measures are within normal limits, however, the response to the fistula test was positive.

IMPRESSION

Left ear fistula with markedly impaired hearing sensitivity.

OUTCOME

Surgical repair of the fistula. Vertigo and balance problems cleared postoperatively, but the hearing loss remained stable. She rejected hearing aid use following a 9-week trial with amplification.

PRESENTING INFORMATION

Pt. states that he has had no use of his left ear "for a long time." He wears a powerful BTE aid on his right ear. He is a poor lipreader. His hx reveals that he is adventitiously deaf, unemployed, and supported by SSI. In addition to deafness, he has several limiting physical and medical conditions.

Impedance measures reveal reduced compliance at normal pressure AU.

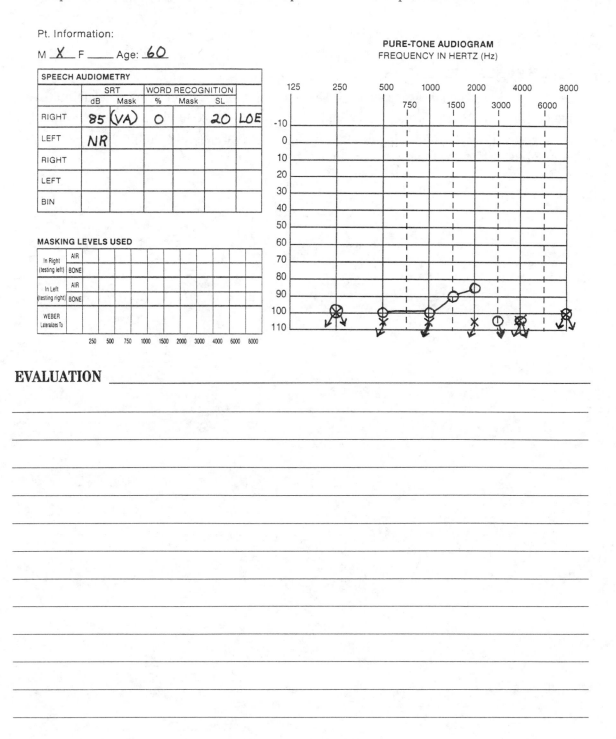

Pt. Information:

M _X_ F ____ Age: _60_

SPEECH AUDIOMETRY

	SRT		WORD RECOGNITION			
	dB	Mask	%	Mask	SL	
RIGHT	85	(VA)	O		20	LOE
LEFT	NR					
RIGHT						
LEFT						
BIN						

MASKING LEVELS USED

In Right (testing left)	AIR									
	BONE									
In Left (testing right)	AIR									
	BONE									
WEBER Lateralizes To										
		250	500	750	1000	1500	2000	3000	4000	6000	8000

PURE-TONE AUDIOGRAM
FREQUENCY IN HERTZ (Hz)

EVALUATION

INTERPRETATION

Auditory assessment reveals a profound SN loss in the left ear and a severe to profound SN loss in the right ear. He has some voice awareness in the right ear but no speech discrimination ability. There is no response to speech testing in the left ear. Both tympanograms reflect borderline-normal compliance at normal middle ear pressure. His lipreading ability is very limited, and he does not appear to benefit from use of his hearing aid.

RECOMMENDATIONS

Referral to a community speech and hearing center for assessment of his rehabilitative needs. He may require formal lipreading lessons, counseling services for the deaf, and assistive devices (pager, TTD, alarm systems etc.). The cochlear implant can not be considered for him due to physical and financial limitations.

PRESENTING INFORMATION

Decreased hearing, greater in right ear. Annoying right ear tinnitus for past 6 months. Normal tympanograms.

Absent acoustic reflex AU.

Pt. Information:

M __X__ F _____ Age: __76__

PURE-TONE AUDIOGRAM
FREQUENCY IN HERTZ (Hz)

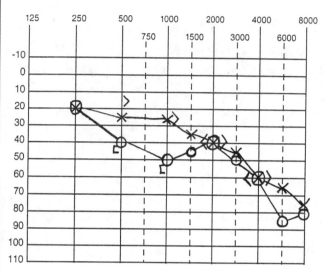

SPEECH AUDIOMETRY						
	SRT		WORD RECOGNITION			
	dB	Mask	%	Mask	SL	
RIGHT	50		92		25	MCL
LEFT	35		84		35	MCL
RIGHT			48	70	40	
LEFT			92	70	55	
BIN						

MASKING LEVELS USED

In Right (testing left)	AIR									
	BONE									
In Left (testing right)	AIR									
	BONE	60	60							
WEBER Lateralizes To										
		250	500	750	1000	1500	2000	3000	4000	6000	8000

EVALUATION _____

_____

_____

_____

_____

_____

_____

_____

_____

_____

_____

_____

_____

INTERPRETATION

Bilateral mild, sloping to severe, SN hearing loss. The loss is asymmetrical in the mid frequencies with the right ear having the greater deficit. Speech discrimination ability with standard presentation is good, right ear, and fairly good, left ear. There is positive PI-PB rollover, however, for the right ear. Both tympanograms are normal. The acoustic reflex is absent bilaterally.

RECOMMENDATIONS

Rule out retrocochlear pathology (based on the asymmetrical loss, positive rollover, and absent acoustic reflex).

PRESENTING INFORMATION

This pt. complains of bilateral hearing loss and tinnitus following completion of Gentamicin treatment.

Both tympanograms are WNL. The acoustic reflex is present with right ear stimulation (with no decay) and is absent with left ear stimulation.

Pt. Information:

M ____ F __X__ Age: __41__

SPEECH AUDIOMETRY

	SRT		WORD RECOGNITION		
	dB	Mask	%	Mask	SL
RIGHT	35		100		30
LEFT	35		100		30
RIGHT					
LEFT					
BIN					

MASKING LEVELS USED

In Right (testing left)	AIR									
	BONE									
In Left (testing right)	AIR									
	BONE									
WEBER Lateralizes To										
		250	500	750	1000	1500	2000	3000	4000	6000	8000

PURE-TONE AUDIOGRAM
FREQUENCY IN HERTZ (Hz)

EVALUATION

_____

_____

_____

_____

_____

_____

_____

_____

_____

_____

_____

_____

_____

INTERPRETATION

Audiologic assessment reveals bilateral mild-moderate essentially SN hearing loss with excellent speech discrimination ability in each ear. Both tympanograms reflect normal middle ear function. The acoustic reflex is absent with left ear stimulation. The reflex is elicited with right ear stimulation and does not decay.

IMPRESSION

Gentamycin ototoxicity.

RECOMMENDATION

Retest in one month to determine the stability of the hearing loss. The test results were explained to the pt., and the recommendation for binaural amplification was made (pending the outcome of the retest). The pt. was lost to follow-up.

PRESENTING INFORMATION

Slight hearing loss in left ear for one year. Hearing loss in right ear for at least 5 years. Frequent otalgia. Cannot tolerate lying on her right side.

No vestibular problems.

Normal middle ear compliance and pressure AU.

The acoustic reflex is absent in the right ear and is present (without decay) in the left ear.

Pt. Information:

M _____ F _X_ Age: **65**

SPEECH AUDIOMETRY

	SRT dB	SRT Mask	WORD RECOGNITION %	WORD RECOGNITION Mask	WORD RECOGNITION SL	
RIGHT	75	55	20	65	15	MCL
LEFT	35		100		35	
RIGHT						
LEFT						
BIN						

MASKING LEVELS USED

In Right (testing left)	AIR									
	BONE									
In Left (testing right)	AIR	65	70	→						
	BONE	65	70	→						
WEBER Lateralizes To										
		250	500	750	1000	1500	2000	3000	4000	6000	8000

PURE-TONE AUDIOGRAM
FREQUENCY IN HERTZ (Hz)

EVALUATION
_____
_____
_____
_____
_____
_____
_____
_____
_____
_____
_____

INTERPRETATION

RIGHT EAR: A severe SN hearing loss with poor speech discrimination ability. The tympanogram is normal; the acoustic reflex is absent.

LEFT EAR: A mild to moderate SN loss with excellent speech discrimination, normal tympanogram, and normal acoustic reflex activity.

OUTCOME

The otologic exam was WNL. The ABR results were WNL AU. The MRI was negative. Dx: Meniere's disease.

PRESENTING INFORMATION

This 89-year-old man is completely blind and has obvious problems hearing and understanding conversational speech. He has never used hearing aids.

Normal middle ear compliance and pressure AU. The acoustic reflex is not elicited AU.

Pt. Information:

M __X__ F ____ Age: __89__

SPEECH AUDIOMETRY

	SRT		WORD RECOGNITION		
	dB	Mask	%	Mask	SL
RIGHT	30		52		30
LEFT	30		52		30
RIGHT					
LEFT					
BIN			56		30

MASKING LEVELS USED

In Right (testing left)	AIR									
	BONE									
In Left (testing right)	AIR									
	BONE									
WEBER Lateralizes To										
		250	500	750	1000	1500	2000	3000	4000	6000	8000

PURE-TONE AUDIOGRAM
FREQUENCY IN HERTZ (Hz)

EVALUATION _____

_____

_____

_____

_____

_____

_____

_____

_____

_____

_____

_____

_____

_____

INTERPRETATION

Bilateral precipitous SN hearing loss (mild, dropping to profound). Speech discrimination scores are reduced in each ear and binaurally. Middle ear compliance and pressure are normal, but there is no acoustic reflex.

RECOMMENDATIONS

Bilateral hearing aids. Because of his financial situation, he is referred to a community speech and hearing center where there is a charitable hearing aid fund for which he is eligible.

PRESENTING INFORMATION

There is a 5-year hx of vertigo accompanied by deteriorating hearing. Radiologic, neurologic, and audiologic tests do not provide a definite diagnosis. She had each ear explored for fistulas. She has been depending on right ear amplification but has not been able to understand speech for the past 6 months. She is a professional woman who is now unable to function satisfactorily at work.

Normal tympanograms. No acoustic reflex.

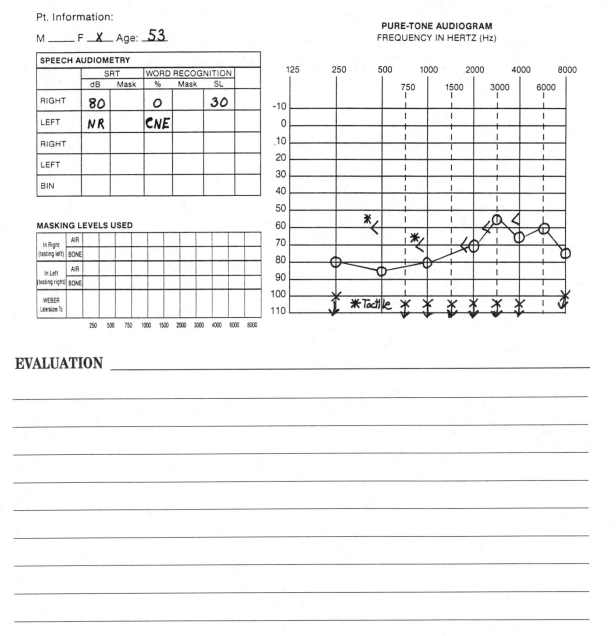

Pt. Information:

M _____ F __X__ Age: __53__

SPEECH AUDIOMETRY

	SRT dB	SRT Mask	WORD RECOGNITION %	WORD RECOGNITION Mask	WORD RECOGNITION SL
RIGHT	80		O		30
LEFT	NR		CNE		
RIGHT					
LEFT					
BIN					

MASKING LEVELS USED

In Right (testing left)	AIR									
	BONE									
In Left (testing right)	AIR									
	BONE									
WEBER Lateralizes To										
		250	500	750	1000	1500	2000	3000	4000	6000	8000

PURE-TONE AUDIOGRAM
FREQUENCY IN HERTZ (Hz)

EVALUATION

INTERPRETATION

There is a severe SN hearing loss with no word discrimination ability in the right ear. There is a profound SN loss in the left ear with no response to pure tone or speech stimuli. Both tympanograms are WNL. There is no acoustic reflex in either ear. Her hearing aid provides only enhanced sound awareness but does not improve speech discrimination.

Her test results suggest that she is now a candidate for the cochlear implant (left ear).

OUTCOME

The cochlear implant evaluation confirmed her eligibility for this surgery. Following implantation, she demonstrated average left ear thresholds of 30 dB with 86% open-set speech discrimination. She has a 72% score on the NU-6 word list. She is able to use the telephone and has returned to work.

PRESENTING INFORMATION

This woman is the victim of spousal abuse. She was beaten, and her left TM was perforated 6 months ago. A SN loss was identified at that time. She did not have the MRI that was scheduled. She now presents with a complaint of mild instability without vertigo. The left TM has healed.

Normal middle ear compliance and pressure AU. The acoustic reflex is present only in the right ear. The results of the Stenger Test (for unilateral nonorganic hearing loss) were negative.

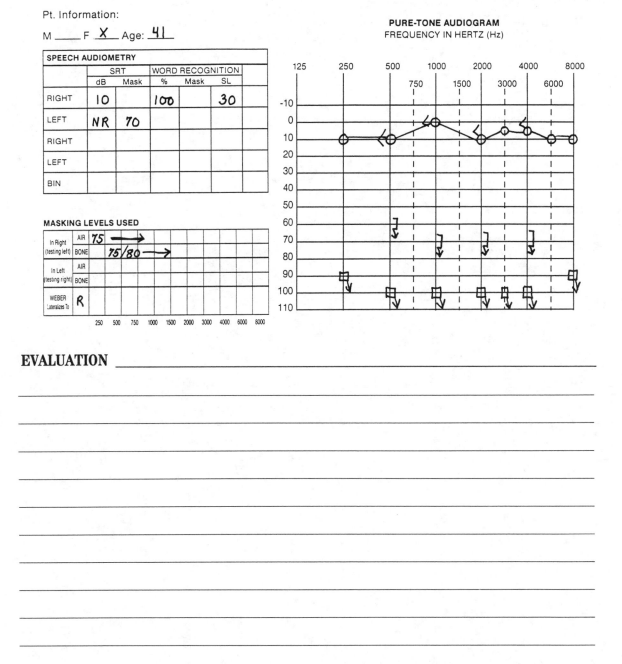

Pt. Information:

M _____ F _X_ Age: _41_

SPEECH AUDIOMETRY

	SRT		WORD RECOGNITION		
	dB	Mask	%	Mask	SL
RIGHT	10		100		30
LEFT	NR	70			
RIGHT					
LEFT					
BIN					

MASKING LEVELS USED

In Right (testing left)	AIR	75 →
	BONE	75/80 →
In Left (testing right)	AIR	
	BONE	
WEBER Lateralizes To	R	

250 500 750 1000 1500 2000 3000 4000 6000 8000

PURE-TONE AUDIOGRAM
FREQUENCY IN HERTZ (Hz)

EVALUATION

_____
_____
_____
_____
_____
_____
_____
_____
_____
_____
_____

INTERPRETATION

Auditory assessment reveals normal hearing sensitivity in the right ear with excellent speech discrimination ability. There is a profound SN loss in the left ear with no word recognition. The Pure Tone Stenger Test results are negative (with no interference and with crossover levels supporting the profundity of the loss). Tympanometry reveals normal middle ear compliance and pressure AU. The acoustic reflex is present only in the right ear.

RECOMMENDATION

Another MRI has been scheduled.

PRESENTING INFORMATION

Pt. had a left mastoidectomy over 10 years ago. He now presents with left otorrhea and otalgia.

Could not test middle ear function (could not seal either ear canal for the test).

Pt. Information:

M _X_ F ____ Age: _58_

PURE-TONE AUDIOGRAM
FREQUENCY IN HERTZ (Hz)

SPEECH AUDIOMETRY

	SRT		WORD RECOGNITION			
	dB	Mask	%	Mask	SL	
RIGHT	5		96		30	
LEFT	70	65	76	75	25	MCL
RIGHT						
LEFT						
BIN						

MASKING LEVELS USED

In Right (testing left)	AIR	80	80		75	→						
	BONE		75/80	→								
In Left (testing right)	AIR											
	BONE											
WEBER Lateralizes To												
		250	500	750	1000	1500	2000	3000	4000	6000	8000	

EVALUATION _____

_____

_____

_____

_____

_____

_____

_____

_____

_____

_____

_____

_____

_____

INTERPRETATION

RIGHT EAR: Mild to moderate SN hearing loss with excellent speech discrimination ability.

LEFT EAR: Severe to profound SN hearing loss, worse in low frequencies. Fair speech discrimination score. Tympanometry could not be accomplished due to inability to establish a seal of either ear canal.

RECOMMENDATION

This pt. appears to be a good candidate for a BICROS hearing aid. A trial with amplification will be arranged when medical clearance for hearing aid use can be provided.

PRESENTING INFORMATION

This 28-year-old woman complains of gradually diminishing hearing in the left ear. She was alarmed when she recently noticed that voices sound like "Donald Duck" in that ear.

Normal middle ear test results AU. The acoustic reflex is present in the right ear. The ipsilateral reflex is present in the left ear, but the contralateral reflex is absent.

There is significant tone decay in the left ear.

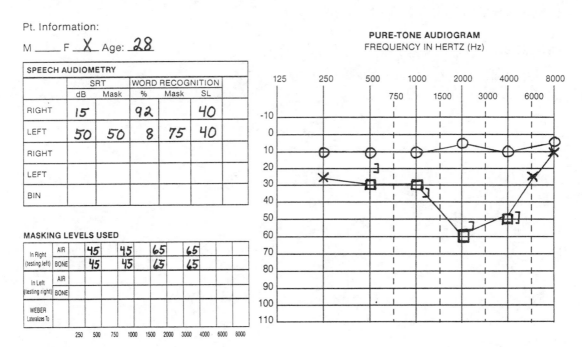

Pt. Information:

M _____ F _X_ Age: _28_

SPEECH AUDIOMETRY

	SRT		WORD RECOGNITION		
	dB	Mask	%	Mask	SL
RIGHT	15		92		40
LEFT	50	50	8	75	40
RIGHT					
LEFT					
BIN					

MASKING LEVELS USED

In Right (testing left)	AIR	45	45	65	65					
	BONE	45	45	65	65					
In Left (testing right)	AIR									
	BONE									
WEBER Lateralizes To										
		250	500	750	1000	1500	2000	3000	4000	6000	8000

PURE-TONE AUDIOGRAM
FREQUENCY IN HERTZ (Hz)

EVALUATION _____

_____

_____

_____

_____

_____

_____

_____

_____

_____

_____

_____

_____

INTERPRETATION

RIGHT EAR: Normal hearing sensitivity with good speech discrimination ability. The acoustic reflex is present.

LEFT EAR: Mild to moderate SN hearing loss which recovers to WNL above 4000 Hz. The speech discrimination score is very poor. The contralateral acoustic reflex is absent with tone left but is present with ipsilateral presentation. A STAT Tone Decay Test revealed rapid decay at 1K, 2K, and 4K Hz.

OUTCOME

A left acoustic neuroma was identified by the MRI.

PRESENTING INFORMATION

Two-year hx of unsteadiness and true vertigo. Sx vary in occurrence and duration. Associated sx include nausea, vomiting, right ear hearing loss, aural fullness, and tinnitus. She has, in the recent past, suffered a heart attack and is taking 6 medications for her cardiovascular problems.

Acoustic impedance measures revealed normal middle ear function AU. The acoustic reflex is elicited AU and does not decay.

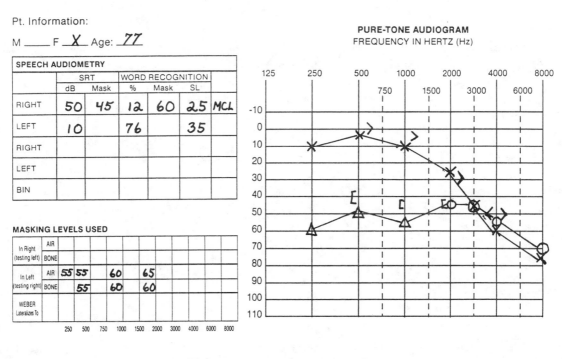

Pt. Information:

M _____ F _X_ Age: _77_

SPEECH AUDIOMETRY

	SRT		WORD RECOGNITION			
	dB	Mask	%	Mask	SL	
RIGHT	50	45	12	60	25	MCL
LEFT	10		76		35	
RIGHT						
LEFT						
BIN						

MASKING LEVELS USED

In Right (testing left)	AIR								
	BONE								
In Left (testing right)	AIR	55	55		60		65		
	BONE		55		60		60		
WEBER Lateralizes To									
		250	500	750	1000	1500	2000	3000	4000	6000	8000

PURE-TONE AUDIOGRAM
FREQUENCY IN HERTZ (Hz)

EVALUATION _____

_____

_____

_____

_____

_____

_____

_____

_____

_____

_____

_____

INTERPRETATION

RIGHT EAR: Moderate SN hearing loss. Poor speech discrimination score.

LEFT EAR: Hearing sensitivity is WNL 250 through 1000 Hz. There is a mild, sloping to profound, high frequency SN loss. Speech discrimination is fair. Middle ear measures are normal, and acoustic reflexes are present without decay AU.

OUTCOME

All diagnostic test results were consistent with the dx of Meniere's disease. A hearing aid evaluation is scheduled.

PRESENTING INFORMATION

SN hearing loss in over 100 family members. He had a mild-moderate loss in childhood, which has progressed. As with other known family members, he has diplacusis, severe recruitment, and has never been able to tolerate amplification. His mother has had a cochlear implant with good results. He uses total communication.

Middle ear pressure and compliance are normal AU. The acoustic reflex is not elicited AU.

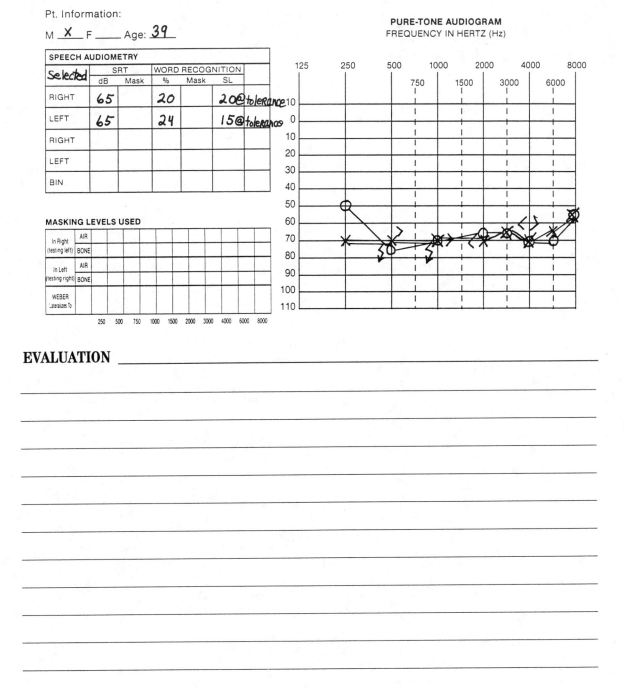

Pt. Information:

M __X__ F _____ Age: __39__

SPEECH AUDIOMETRY

Selected	SRT		WORD RECOGNITION		
	dB	Mask	%	Mask	SL
RIGHT	65		20		20@tolerance
LEFT	65		24		15@tolerance
RIGHT					
LEFT					
BIN					

MASKING LEVELS USED

In Right (testing left)	AIR								
	BONE								
In Left (testing right)	AIR								
	BONE								
WEBER Lateralizes To									
		250	500	750	1000	1500	2000	3000	4000	6000	8000

PURE-TONE AUDIOGRAM
FREQUENCY IN HERTZ (Hz)

EVALUATION _____

_____

_____

_____

_____

_____

_____

_____

_____

_____

_____

_____

_____

INTERPRETATION

Auditory assessment reveals bilateral severe SN hearing loss with poor speech discrimination. The loss is also characterized by a severe tolerance problem (which limited the presentation level of the speech discrimination tests). Middle ear measurements are normal. The acoustic reflex is absent AU.

RECOMMENDATIONS

Trial with computer selected and governed hearing aids. Annual monitoring of hearing loss. He is not now a candidate for the cochlear implant as his hearing thresholds are outside the current FDA guidelines for implantation.

SECTION 2

CONDUCTIVE HEARING LOSS

PRESENTING INFORMATION

CC: Hearing loss L > R. Sixteen-year-old unrestrained driver in MVA sustained left parietal open and depressed skull fx together with orthopedic and intra-abdominal injuries. Pt. now c/o left hearing loss but denies tinnitus or vertigo. No facial nerve deficit.

MIDDLE EAR MEASURES		RIGHT	LEFT
	ECV:	1.2 ml	1.5 ml
	COMP:	.2 ml	.1 ml
	MEP:	-100 daPa	Flat

Pt. Information:

M _X_ F ____ Age: _16_

PURE-TONE AUDIOGRAM
FREQUENCY IN HERTZ (Hz)

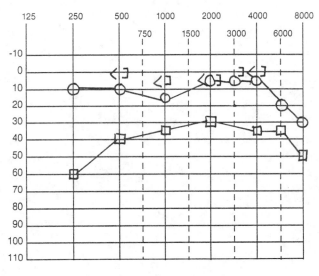

SPEECH AUDIOMETRY

	SRT		WORD RECOGNITION		
	dB	Mask	%	Mask	SL
RIGHT	10		96		30
LEFT	35		96	55	30
RIGHT					
LEFT					
BIN					

MASKING LEVELS USED

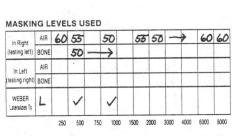

In Right (testing left)	AIR	60	55	50		55	50	→	60	60
	BONE		50	→						
In Left (testing right)	AIR									
	BONE									
WEBER Lateralizes To	L		✓		✓					

250 500 750 1000 1500 2000 3000 4000 6000 8000

EVALUATION _____

_____

_____

_____

_____

_____

_____

_____

_____

_____

_____

INTERPRETATION

RIGHT EAR: Essentially normal hearing sensitivity except for a mild deficit at 6 and 8 KHz. The tympanogram, however, reflects reduced ME compliance at slightly negative pressure.

LEFT EAR: Mild-moderate conductive loss with excellent word discrimination ability. There is a non compliant ME system.

OUTCOME

Left canal debridement. Left hemotympanum. Temporal bone CT was ordered although fx was not considered likely.

PRESENTING INFORMATION:

Pt. was hit in the head with a board. Basilar skull fx. Required right facial nerve decompression. Now presenting with complete right VIIth nerve degeneration.

MIDDLE EAR MEASURES:	RIGHT	LEFT
ECV:	1.7 ml	1.5 ml
COMP:	0 ml	1.0 ml
MEP:	Flat	0 daPa

Pt. Information:

M _X_ F ____ Age: **47**

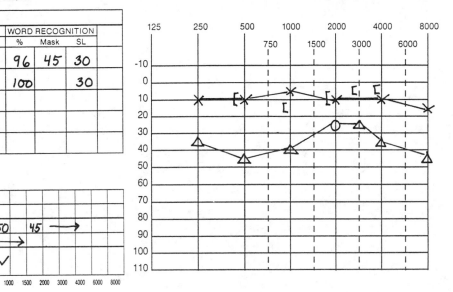

SPEECH AUDIOMETRY

	SRT dB	SRT Mask	WORD RECOGNITION %	WORD RECOGNITION Mask	WORD RECOGNITION SL
RIGHT	25	40	96	45	30
LEFT	5		100		30
RIGHT					
LEFT					
BIN					

MASKING LEVELS USED

		250	500	750	1000	1500	2000	3000	4000	6000	8000
In Right (testing left)	AIR										
	BONE										
In Left (testing right)	AIR	45	50		50		45	→			
	BONE		50	→	→						
WEBER Lateralizes To	R	✓		✓							

EVALUATION _____

_____

_____

_____

_____

_____

_____

_____

_____

_____

_____

_____

INTERPRETATION

RIGHT EAR: Mild conductive hearing loss with very good word discrimination. Abnormal (noncompliant) middle ear system.

LEFT EAR: Normal hearing sensitivity, word discrimination, and middle ear function.

PRESENTING INFORMATION

Hx of recurrent serous otitis media. Radiologic confirmation of tumor in the nasopharynx.

MIDDLE EAR MEASURES:		RIGHT	LEFT
	ECV:	1.3 ml	1.4 ml
	COMP:	0 ml	0 ml
	MEP:	Flat	Flat

Pt. Information:

M _____ F _X_ Age: _67_

SPEECH AUDIOMETRY

	SRT		WORD RECOGNITION		
	dB	Mask	%	Mask	SL
RIGHT	25		100		30
LEFT	20		100		30
RIGHT					
LEFT					
BIN					

PURE-TONE AUDIOGRAM
FREQUENCY IN HERTZ (Hz)

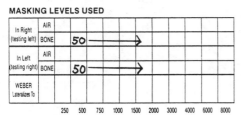

MASKING LEVELS USED

In Right (testing left)	AIR									
	BONE	50 →								
In Left (testing right)	AIR									
	BONE	50 →								
WEBER Lateralizes To										

250   500   750   1000   1500   2000   3000   4000   6000   8000

EVALUATION _____

_____

_____

_____

_____

_____

_____

_____

_____

_____

_____

INTERPRETATION

Mild-to-moderate conductive hearing loss, bilaterally. Speech discrimination is excellent in each ear. Tympanometry reveals noncompliant middle ear systems at normal physical volume.

PRESENTING INFORMATION

Pt. jammed toothpick through his left tympanic membrane 3 days ago. His cc is throbbing pain in the left ear.

MIDDLE EAR MEASURES:

	RIGHT	LEFT
ECV:	1.8 ml	1.2 ml
COMP:	1.0 ml	0 ml
MEP:	+40 daPa	Flat

Pt. Information:

M __X__ F _____ Age: __41__

SPEECH AUDIOMETRY

	SRT		WORD RECOGNITION		
	dB	Mask	%	Mask	SL
RIGHT	5		100		35
LEFT	30	45	96	45	30
RIGHT					
LEFT					
BIN					

MASKING LEVELS USED

In Right (testing left)	AIR	50 →								
	BONE	50 →								
In Left (testing right)	AIR									
	BONE									
WEBER Lateralizes To	L	✓	✓							
	250	500	750	1000	1500	2000	3000	4000	6000	8000

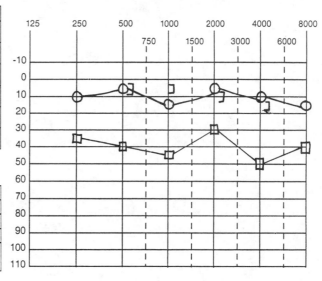

PURE-TONE AUDIOGRAM
FREQUENCY IN HERTZ (Hz)

EVALUATION

_____

_____

_____

_____

_____

_____

_____

_____

_____

_____

INTERPRETATION

RIGHT EAR: Hearing sensitivity is within normal limits. The tympanogram is normal.

LEFT EAR: Moderate conductive hearing loss. 30-40 dB air-bone gap. The tympanogram is flat at normal physical volume.

OUTCOME

Treated for otitis media. Traumatic injury to the middle ear has not been ruled out.

PRESENTING INFORMATION

Pt. had noticed diminished hearing for several months. Last week, while eating a bagel, she suddenly "went deaf" in her right ear.

MIDDLE EAR MEASURES:

	RIGHT	LEFT
ECV:	.5 ml	1.1 ml
COMP:	0 ml	.3 ml
MEP:	Flat	-30 daPa

Pt. Information:

M _____ F **X** Age: **55**

SPEECH AUDIOMETRY

	SRT		WORD RECOGNITION		
	dB	Mask	%	Mask	SL
RIGHT	30		100	55	30
LEFT	10		100		30
RIGHT					
LEFT					
BIN					

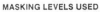

MASKING LEVELS USED

In Right (testing left) AIR									
BONE	55	60	65 →						
In Left (testing right) AIR	40		50	60 →			65	70	
BONE	45	45	50		45				
WEBER Lateralizes To	R	✓	✓						

250 500 750 1000 1500 2000 3000 4000 6000 8000

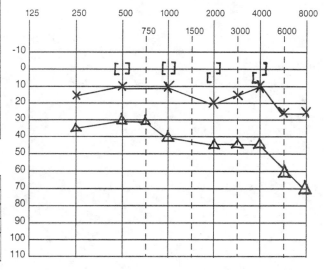

PURE-TONE AUDIOGRAM
FREQUENCY IN HERTZ (Hz)

EVALUATION _____

_____

_____

_____

_____

_____

_____

_____

_____

_____

_____

INTERPRETATION

RIGHT EAR: Mild-to-moderately severe conductive hearing loss. Excellent word discrimination. Weber to right. Flat tympanogram with reduced physical volume. Occluding cerumen.

LEFT EAR: Hearing sensitivity is within normal limits with a small air-bone gap. Excellent discrimination score. The tympanogram is normal although there is excessive cerumen in the canal.

ENT NOTE

Impacted cerumen removed from right ear. Left ear cerumen cleared.

PRESENTING INFORMATION

CC: Left ear hearing loss since childhood. Hx of previous (29 years ago) mastoid surgery on left ear with no documented ossicular repair. Right ear loss of recent onset. Increased adenoid tissue noted in nasopharynx. A CT scan through the neck and an audiologic assessment were ordered.

MIDDLE EAR MEASURES:	RIGHT	LEFT
MEV:	1.7 ml	2.4 ml
COMP:	.1 ml	.1 ml
MEP:	Flat	Flat

Pt. Information:

M _____ F X Age: 47

PURE-TONE AUDIOGRAM
FREQUENCY IN HERTZ (Hz)

SPEECH AUDIOMETRY

	SRT		WORD RECOGNITION		
	dB	Mask	%	Mask	SL
RIGHT	35		96		30
LEFT	55	60	96	75	30
RIGHT					
LEFT					
BIN					

MASKING LEVELS USED

In Right (testing left)	AIR	70	→			70		
	BONE	70	→					
In Left (testing right)	AIR							
	BONE	75	75	65	75			
WEBER Lateralizes To								

250 500 750 1000 1500 2000 3000 4000 6000 8000

EVALUATION _____

_____

_____

_____

_____

_____

_____

_____

_____

_____

INTERPRETATION

RIGHT EAR: Mild conductive hearing loss. Hypocompliant middle ear system with normal physical volume.

LEFT EAR: Moderate to moderately-severe essentially conductive loss (sensorineural component at 4 K Hz). The flat tympanogram with a large physical volume confirms TM perforation.

ENT NOTE

Right SOM likely due to eustachian tube dysfunction. Left TM with dry posterior inferior perforation, fibrous stranding. Malleus and stapes seen, but no incus identified. Tympanotomy and ossiculoplasty/ tympanoplasty recommended.

PRESENTING INFORMATION

Three-month postoperative follow-up of patient who has had left ear ossiculoplasty for fibrous union of the incus to the stapes. She is complaining now of sharp pain in the right TMJ region and locking, clicking jaw. The pt. experienced vertigo during right tympanometry.

MIDDLE EAR MEASURES:	RIGHT	LEFT
ECV:	1.6 ml	1.4 ml
COMP:	.5 ml	1.8 ml
MEP:	-20 daPa	-90 daPa

Pt. Information:

M _____ F _X_ Age: _21_

PURE-TONE AUDIOGRAM
FREQUENCY IN HERTZ (Hz)

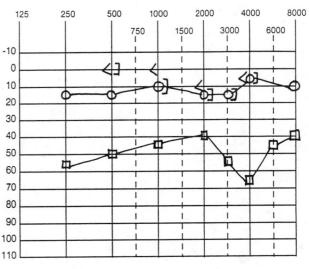

SPEECH AUDIOMETRY

	SRT		WORD RECOGNITION		
	dB	Mask	%	Mask	SL
RIGHT	10		100		30
LEFT	40	45	100	55	30
RIGHT					
LEFT					
BIN					

MASKING LEVELS USED

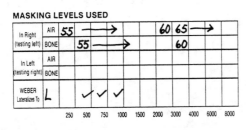

In Right (testing left)	AIR	55	→			60	65	→
	BONE		55	→			60	
In Left (testing right)	AIR							
	BONE							
WEBER Lateralizes To	L	✓	✓	✓				

250 500 750 1000 1500 2000 3000 4000 6000 8000

EVALUATION _____

_____

_____

_____

_____

_____

_____

_____

_____

_____

INTERPRETATION

RIGHT EAR: Normal hearing sensitivity. Normal tympanogram. Spontaneous report of dizziness during impedance test. Repeated test with eyes closed caused dizziness to increase. Rule out fistula.

LEFT EAR: Moderate-severe conductive loss which is similar to preoperative audiogram. Tympanometry reveals a hypercompliant middle ear system at slightly negative pressure.

OUTCOME

Patient was treated for TMJ dysfunction.

PRESENTING INFORMATION

Left ear tympanoplasty 3 months ago. Pt. states that he can hear with the left ear, but all sound is "fuzzy." The TM is well visualized. No pain, no drainage, no erythema. The preoperative audiogram revealed a flat, average 40 dB left ear conductive loss.

MIDDLE EAR MEASURES:	RIGHT	LEFT
ECV:	1.5 ml	1.7 ml
COMP:	.5 ml	0 ml
MEP:	-20 daPa	Flat

Pt. Information:

M _X_ F _____ Age: _35_

SPEECH AUDIOMETRY

	SRT		WORD RECOGNITION		
	dB	Mask	%	Mask	SL
RIGHT	10		96		30
LEFT	25		96	50	30
RIGHT					
LEFT					
BIN					

MASKING LEVELS USED

In Right (testing left)	AIR	50 →								
	BONE	50 →								
In Left (testing right)	AIR									
	BONE									
WEBER Lateralizes To	L			✓	✓					
	250	500	750	1000	1500	2000	3000	4000	6000	8000

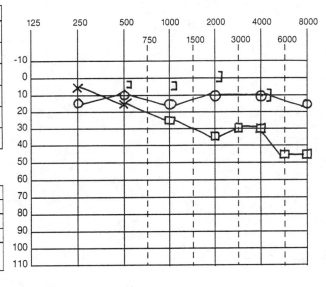

PURE-TONE AUDIOGRAM
FREQUENCY IN HERTZ (Hz)

EVALUATION _____

_____

_____

_____

_____

_____

_____

_____

_____

_____

_____

INTERPRETATION

RIGHT EAR: Normal audiogram and tympanogram.

LEFT EAR: Normal low frequency hearing with a mild conductive loss above 500 Hz. (Hearing sensitivity has improved since the preoperative tests as the result of the complete or partial closure of the air-bone gap through low and mid frequencies.) The speech discrimination score is very good. The tympanogram is flat at normal physical volume.

RECOMMENDATION

Retest at 3-month intervals (sooner if there are problems or complications).

PRESENTING INFORMATION

CC: Right ear had clear running discharge last week. Longstanding right TM perforation. Fifty percent inferior central perforation. Remaining TM is sclerotic. No drainage seen. Vague complaint of dizziness.

MIDDLE EAR MEASURES:		RIGHT	LEFT
	MEV:	5.2 ml	1.7 ml
	COMP:	0 ml	1.4 ml
	MEP:	Flat	-10 daPa

Pt. Information:

M ____ F __X__ Age: __62__

SPEECH AUDIOMETRY

	SRT dB	SRT Mask	WORD RECOGNITION %	WORD RECOGNITION Mask	WORD RECOGNITION SL
RIGHT	55	45	96	55	30
LEFT	5		100		30
RIGHT					
LEFT					
BIN					

MASKING LEVELS USED

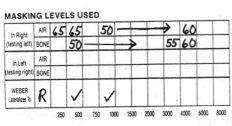

In Right (testing left)	AIR	65	65	50	→		60	
	BONE		50	→	→		55	60
In Left (testing right)	AIR							
	BONE							
WEBER Lateralizes To	R	✓		✓				

250 500 750 1000 1500 2000 3000 4000 6000 8000

PURE-TONE AUDIOGRAM
FREQUENCY IN HERTZ (Hz)

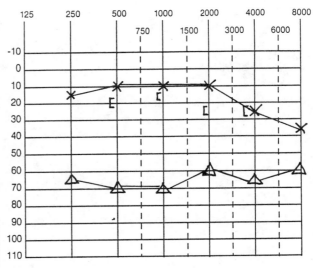

EVALUATION _____

_____

_____

_____

_____

_____

_____

_____

_____

_____

INTERPRETATION

RIGHT EAR: Severe conductive hearing loss with excellent word discrimination score. There is a large physical volume per tympanometry, which is consistent with the TM perforation.

LEFT EAR: Normal hearing thresholds 250 through 4000 Hz with a mild deficit at 8K Hz. Word discrimination is excellent. The tympanogram revealed normal middle ear function.

OUTCOME

A tympanoplasty and ossiculoplasty was recommended by the physician.

PRESENTING INFORMATION:

Pt. with AIDS-related complications. His cc is tinnitus.

MIDDLE EAR MEASURES:	RIGHT	LEFT
ECV:	1.3 ml	1.5 ml
COMP:	1.1 ml	.9 ml
MEP:	-48 daPa	-24 daPa

Pt. Information:

M __X__ F _____ Age: __25__

SPEECH AUDIOMETRY

	SRT		WORD RECOGNITION		
	dB	Mask	%	Mask	SL
RIGHT	5		96		30
LEFT	5		96		30
RIGHT					
LEFT					
BIN					

MASKING LEVELS USED

In Right (testing left)	AIR									
	BONE									
In Left (testing right)	AIR									
	BONE	50 →			45 →					
WEBER Lateralizes To	R		✓							
		250	500	750	1000	1500	2000	3000	4000	6000	8000

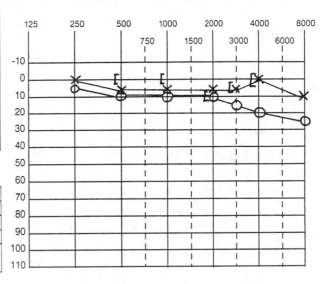

PURE-TONE AUDIOGRAM
FREQUENCY IN HERTZ (Hz)

EVALUATION _____

_____

_____

_____

_____

_____

_____

_____

_____

_____

_____

_____

_____

INTERPRETATION

Bilateral normal hearing sensitivity characterized by a mild conductive reduction in right ear hearing thresholds at the high frequencies. Speech detection and discrimination scores are normal. Both tympanograms reflect normal middle ear function. The acoustic reflex is elicited AU.

OUTCOME

The physician reported that there is otitis externa (fungus) in each ear canal. Treatment was prescribed, and patient was advised to return if his tinnitus did not improve.

PRESENTING INFORMATION

This young man was attacked and beaten 4 days ago. He has sustained jaw and facial injuries. He also complains of hearing loss in the right ear. His face and right pinna are swollen and bruised, but there is no blood in the ear canal.

MIDDLE EAR MEASURES:

	RIGHT	LEFT
MEV:	1.4 ml	2.5 ml
COMP:	.6 ml	1.3 ml
MEP:	+18 daPa	-20 daPa
ACOUSTIC REFLEX:	Present	Absent

Pt. Information:

M _X_ F ____ Age: **24**

SPEECH AUDIOMETRY

	SRT		WORD RECOGNITION		
	dB	Mask	%	Mask	SL
RIGHT	40	45	100	55	30
LEFT	5		100		30
RIGHT					
LEFT					
BIN					

MASKING LEVELS USED

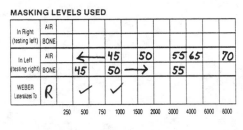

In Right (testing left)	AIR							
	BONE							
In Left (testing right)	AIR	←	45	50		55	65	70
	BONE	45	50	→		55		
WEBER Lateralizes To	R	✓		✓				

250 500 750 1000 1500 2000 3000 4000 6000 8000

PURE-TONE AUDIOGRAM
FREQUENCY IN HERTZ (Hz)

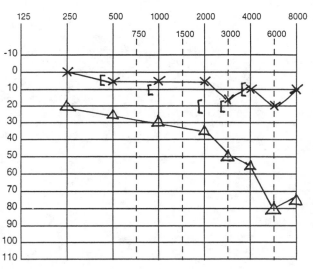

EVALUATION _____

_____

_____

_____

_____

_____

_____

_____

_____

_____

INTERPRETATION

RIGHT EAR: The Weber refers to the right ear, and there is a mild to severe, sloping, conductive loss. The tympanogram appears unusual, yet values are WNL. A repeated test also showed the same pattern. Rule out ossicular discontinuity.

LEFT EAR: Normal audiogram, speech scores, and middle ear function. The acoustic reflex is elicited.

OUTCOME

After the pt. was released from the hospital, he did not return for follow-up.

PRESENTING INFORMATION

Pt. is 27 weeks pregnant and presents with right ear pain and decreased hearing for last 7 weeks. Treated for sinus infection 4 weeks prior to the onset of the ear symptoms. The nasal discharge cleared with treatment but hearing diminished.

MIDDLE EAR MEASURES:	LEFT	RIGHT
MEV:	1.6 ml	1.4 ml
COMP:	.3 ml	0 ml
MEP:	-10 daPa	Flat

Pt. Information:

M _____ F **X** Age: **38**

SPEECH AUDIOMETRY

	SRT		WORD RECOGNITION		
	dB	Mask	%	Mask	SL
RIGHT	40	45	100	65	30
LEFT	5		100		30
RIGHT					
LEFT					
BIN					

MASKING LEVELS USED

		250	500	750	1000	1500	2000	3000	4000	6000	8000
In Right (testing left)	AIR										
	BONE										
In Left (testing right)	AIR	55	60		55		50	55	70 →		
	BONE		60 →						70		
WEBER Lateralizes To	R	✓		✓							

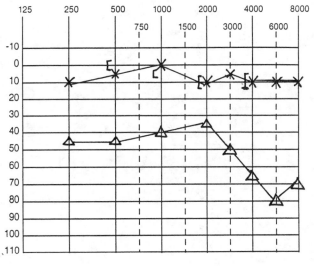

PURE-TONE AUDIOGRAM
FREQUENCY IN HERTZ (Hz)

EVALUATION

_____

_____

_____

_____

_____

_____

_____

_____

_____

_____

_____

INTERPRETATION

RIGHT EAR: Mild to severe conductive hearing loss with excellent word discrimination. There is no measured compliance of the middle ear system.

LEFT EAR: Normal hearing sensitivity with normal middle ear compliance and pressure.

DIAGNOSIS

Otitis media, right ear.

PRESENTING INFORMATION

Pt. with advanced AIDS presents with cc of left ear hearing loss. Left ear is draining.

MIDDLE EAR MEASURES:

	RIGHT	LEFT
MEV:	2.4 ml	CNT
COMP:	.5 ml	
MEP:	-30 daPa	

Pt. Information:

M _X_ F ____ Age: _36_

SPEECH AUDIOMETRY

	SRT dB	SRT Mask	WORD RECOGNITION %	WORD RECOGNITION Mask	WORD RECOGNITION SL
RIGHT	10		96		30
LEFT	35		96	60	30
RIGHT					
LEFT					
BIN					

MASKING LEVELS USED

		250	500	750	1000	1500	2000	3000	4000	6000	8000
In Right (testing left)	AIR	50	60	→						70	70
In Right (testing left)	BONE	65	→								
In Left (testing right)	AIR										
In Left (testing right)	BONE										
WEBER Lateralizes To	L	✓									

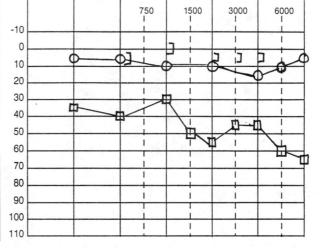

PURE-TONE AUDIOGRAM
FREQUENCY IN HERTZ (Hz)

EVALUATION

_____

_____

_____

_____

_____

_____

_____

_____

_____

_____

INTERPRETATION

RIGHT EAR: Normal hearing sensitivity, speech discrimination, and middle ear function.

LEFT EAR: Mild-moderate conductive hearing loss. Very good speech discrimination score. Could not evaluate middle ear function due to discharge from ear.

DIAGNOSIS

Swollen ear canal with copious discharge. Otitis externa.

PRESENTING INFORMATION:

Morbidly obese pt. with hx of right tympanomastoid surgery 8 years ago. Now presenting with complaint of progressing bilateral hearing loss.

MIDDLE EAR MEASURES:

	RIGHT	LEFT
MEV:	2.0 ml	1.4 ml
COMP:	0 ml	0 ml
MEP:	Flat	Flat

Pt. Information:

M __X__ F _____ Age: __30__

SPEECH AUDIOMETRY

	SRT dB	SRT Mask	WORD RECOGNITION %	WORD RECOGNITION Mask	SL
RIGHT	30		100		30
LEFT	50	50	100	70	30
RIGHT					
LEFT					
BIN					

MASKING LEVELS USED

In Right (testing left) AIR	80	75	75	70	→					75
In Right (testing left) BONE	75	75	75	70	→					
In Left (testing right) AIR										
In Left (testing right) BONE	80	80		75/80	→					
WEBER Lateralizes To										

250 500 750 1000 1500 2000 3000 4000 6000 8000

PURE-TONE AUDIOGRAM
FREQUENCY IN HERTZ (Hz)

EVALUATION _____

_____

_____

_____

_____

_____

_____

_____

_____

_____

_____

INTERPRETATION

RIGHT EAR: Mild, essentially conductive hearing loss. Flat tympanogram with increased physical volume (significant TM retraction).

LEFT EAR: Moderate, essentially conductive hearing loss. Flat tympanogram with normal physical volume. Both ears have excellent word discrimination scores - consistent with the nature of the hearing loss.

DIAGNOSIS

Chronic otitis media.

PRESENTING INFORMATION

Pt. has recently recovered from bronchial pneumonia. She now is experiencing diminished hearing, vertigo, "staggering," and full feeling AU. She is currently receiving therapy for anxiety attacks.

MIDDLE EAR MEASURES:

	RIGHT	LEFT
MEV:	.9 ml	1.1 ml
COMP:	0 ml	0 ml
MEP:	Flat	Flat

Pt. Information:

M _____ F _X_ Age: _29_

SPEECH AUDIOMETRY

	SRT		WORD RECOGNITION		
	dB	Mask	%	Mask	SL
RIGHT	10		96		30
LEFT	15		100	45	30
RIGHT					
LEFT					
BIN					

MASKING LEVELS USED

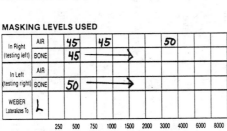

In Right (testing left)	AIR	45	45		50				
	BONE	45	→						
In Left (testing right)	AIR								
	BONE	50	→						
WEBER Lateralizes To	L								

250 500 750 1000 1500 2000 3000 4000 6000 8000

PURE-TONE AUDIOGRAM
FREQUENCY IN HERTZ (Hz)

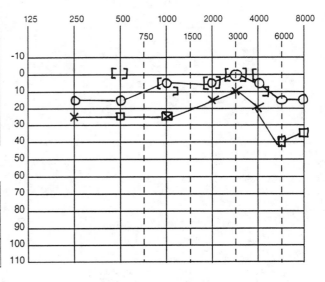

EVALUATION
_____
_____
_____
_____
_____
_____
_____
_____
_____
_____
_____

INTERPRETATION

Right ear hearing sensitivity is normal, but there is a significant low frequency air-bone gap. There is a mild conductive hearing loss in the left ear. Both ears have excellent word discrimination ability.

Tympanometry reveals bilateral noncompliant middle ear systems.

DIAGNOSIS

Bilateral otitis media.

PRESENTING INFORMATION

Annual evaluation of pt. who had right mastoidectomy for cholesteatoma 5 years ago.

MIDDLE EAR MEASURES:	RIGHT	LEFT
ECV:	1.3 ml	1.8 ml
COMP:	0 ml	1.0 ml
MEP:	Flat	-24 daPa

Pt. Information:

M _X_ F _____ Age: _35_

SPEECH AUDIOMETRY

	SRT dB	SRT Mask	WORD RECOGNITION %	WORD RECOGNITION Mask	SL	
RIGHT	65	60	96	75	30	
LEFT	5		96		30	
RIGHT						
LEFT						
BIN						

PURE-TONE AUDIOGRAM
FREQUENCY IN HERTZ (Hz)

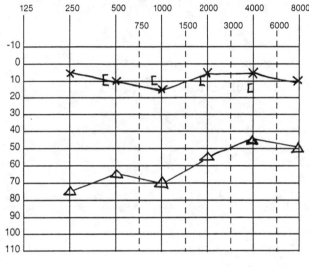

MASKING LEVELS USED

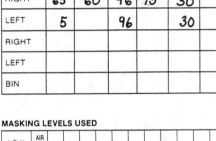

		250	500	750	1000	1500	2000	3000	4000	6000	8000
In Right (testing left)	AIR										
	BONE										
In Left (testing right)	AIR	65	60	→			55	→			
	BONE	55	→								
WEBER Lateralizes To	R	✓		✓							

EVALUATION _____

_____

_____

_____

_____

_____

_____

_____

_____

_____

_____

_____

_____

INTERPRETATION

RIGHT EAR: Moderate-severe conductive hearing loss with excellent speech discrimination. Air conduction thresholds 250 through 1K Hz have increased +25-30 dB since his postoperative test 5 years ago. The tympanogram is flat at normal physical volume.

LEFT EAR: Normal hearing thresholds with normal hearing for speech and normal middle ear function.

RECOMMENDATION

Consider right ear amplification when medical clearance can be given. Use of left ear hearing protection in noise was discussed with him.

DIAGNOSIS

Returning cholesteatoma.

PRESENTING INFORMATION

Fifty two-year-old male with recurrent squamous cell ca of tonsil/neck here for pre-chemotherapy audiogram.

MIDDLE EAR MEASURES:	RIGHT	LEFT
ECV:	1.4 ml	1.5 ml
COMP:	.7 ml	0 ml
MEP:	-42 daPa	Flat

Pt. Information:

M _X_ F _____ Age: _52_

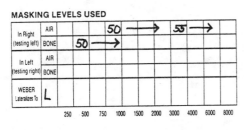

SPEECH AUDIOMETRY

	SRT		WORD RECOGNITION		
	dB	Mask	%	Mask	SL
RIGHT	5		100		30
LEFT	20		100	45	30
RIGHT					
LEFT					
BIN					

MASKING LEVELS USED

In Right (testing left)	AIR			50 →		55 →	
	BONE		50 →				
In Left (testing right)	AIR						
	BONE						
WEBER Lateralizes To	L						

250 500 750 1000 1500 2000 3000 4000 6000 8000

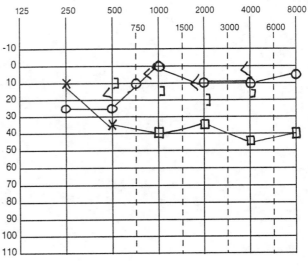

PURE-TONE AUDIOGRAM
FREQUENCY IN HERTZ (Hz)

EVALUATION _____

_____

_____

_____

_____

_____

_____

_____

_____

_____

_____

INTERPRETATION

RIGHT EAR: Normal hearing sensitivity and word discrimination. Normal tympanogram.

LEFT EAR: Mild-to-moderate essentially conductive hearing loss. Weber refers to left. Flat tympanogram at normal physical volume.

DIAGNOSIS

Eustachian tube dysfunction secondary to SCCA/surgery. Recommended PE tube, but pt. was not interested at this time.

PRESENTING INFORMATION

Pt. was accosted with a lead pipe 48 hours ago. Blows were to the back of head and above the left ear.

MIDDLE EAR MEASURES:

	RIGHT	LEFT
ECV:	1.0 ml	1.3 ml
COMP:	1.7 ml	1.3 ml
MEP:	-180 daPa	-300 daPa

ACOUSTIC REFLEX ABSENT AU

Pt. Information:

M _X_ F ____ Age: _38_

SPEECH AUDIOMETRY

	SRT		WORD RECOGNITION		
	dB	Mask	%	Mask	SL
RIGHT	15		100		30
LEFT	25	40	100	50	30
RIGHT					
LEFT					
BIN					

MASKING LEVELS USED

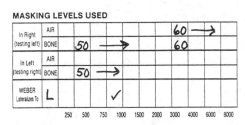

								60 →	
In Right (testing left)	AIR								
	BONE	50	→				60		
In Left (testing right)	AIR								
	BONE	50	→						
WEBER Lateralizes To	L		✓						

250 500 750 1000 1500 2000 3000 4000 6000 8000

PURE-TONE AUDIOGRAM
FREQUENCY IN HERTZ (Hz)

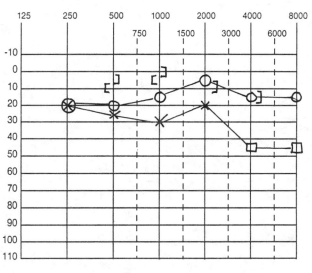

EVALUATION _____

_____

_____

_____

_____

_____

_____

_____

_____

_____

INTERPRETATION

RIGHT EAR: Essentially normal hearing (with a mild deficit below 1K Hz). Excellent word discrimination. Negative middle ear pressure but normal compliance of the system.

LEFT EAR: Mild-to-moderate conductive hearing loss. Weber refers to left. Significantly negative middle ear pressure, but compliance is WNL.

The acoustic reflex is absent AU.

OUTCOME

Hearing sensitivity recovered to WNL in 6 weeks. Tympanograms on retest were normal. The acoustic reflex was present.

PRESENTING INFORMATION

Pt. fell down full flight of stairs 4 weeks ago and sustained head and orthopedic injuries. She has a 70% perforation (anterior) of the left TM. Middle ear is dry.

MIDDLE EAR MEASURES:	RIGHT	LEFT
ECV:	.9 ml	CNT
COMP:	.4 ml	
MEP:	-100 daPa	

Pt. Information:

M _____ F _X_ Age: _18_

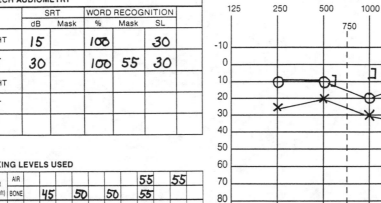

PURE-TONE AUDIOGRAM
FREQUENCY IN HERTZ (Hz)

SPEECH AUDIOMETRY

	SRT		WORD RECOGNITION		
	dB	Mask	%	Mask	SL
RIGHT	15		100		30
LEFT	30		100	55	30
RIGHT					
LEFT					
BIN					

MASKING LEVELS USED

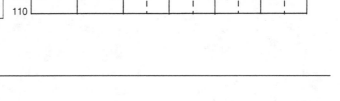

								55	55
In Right (testing left)	AIR							55	55
	BONE		45	50	50	55			
In Left (testing right)	AIR								
	BONE								
WEBER Lateralizes To	L				✓				

250 500 750 1000 1500 2000 3000 4000 6000 8000

EVALUATION _____

_____

_____

_____

_____

_____

_____

_____

_____

_____

_____

INTERPRETATION

RIGHT EAR: Hearing thresholds are WNL. Word discrimination is excellent. Middle ear compliance is normal at mildly negative pressure.

LEFT EAR: Mild to moderate conductive hearing loss with excellent word discrimination. Weber refers to this ear. Could not obtain an effective seal to permit tympanometry.

OUTCOME

Tympanoplasty scheduled for left ear.

PRESENTING INFORMATION

Pt. complains of significant left ear hearing loss. She had tympanomastoid surgery on this ear 2 years ago.

MIDDLE EAR MEASURES:

	RIGHT	LEFT
ECV:	1.7 ml	1.8 ml
COMP:	.6 ml	.1 ml
MEP:	-60 daPa	Flat

Pt. Information:

M _____ F _X_ Age: _32_

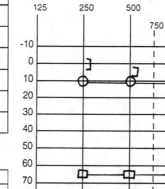

PURE-TONE AUDIOGRAM
FREQUENCY IN HERTZ (Hz)

SPEECH AUDIOMETRY

	SRT		WORD RECOGNITION		
	dB	Mask	%	Mask	SL
RIGHT	10		100		30
LEFT	65	50	100	65	30
RIGHT					
LEFT					
BIN					

MASKING LEVELS USED

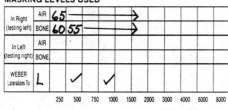

In Right (testing left)	AIR	65	→							
	BONE	60 55	→							
In Left (testing right)	AIR									
	BONE									
WEBER Lateralizes To	L	✓		✓						

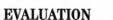

EVALUATION _____

INTERPRETATION

RIGHT EAR: Essentially normal hearing sensitivity (except for a mild deficit at 8K Hz). Excellent discrimination score. Very slightly negative ME pressure with normal compliance.

LEFT EAR: Moderately-severe conductive loss characterized by a "Carhart Notch." Tympanometry reveals a noncompliant middle ear system with normal physical volume.

RECOMMENDATION

Consideration of amplification for the left ear when medical procedures have been completed, and there are no contraindications for hearing aid use.

SECTION 3
MIXED HEARING LOSS

PRESENTING INFORMATION

Hospital inpatient who suffered burns and traumatic injuries when struck by lightning. He is complaining of pain and drainage in the right ear and hearing loss AU. There is a right tympanic membrane perforation and left hemotympanum (puncture hemorrhage).

MIDDLE EAR MEASURES:

	RIGHT	LEFT
MEV:	CNT	1.6 ml
COMP:		.8 ml
MEP:		0 daPa

Pt. Information:

M **X** F _____ Age: **41**

SPEECH AUDIOMETRY

	SRT		WORD RECOGNITION		
	dB	Mask	%	Mask	SL
RIGHT	35	45	76	50	35
LEFT	20		72		35
RIGHT					
LEFT					
BIN					

MASKING LEVELS USED

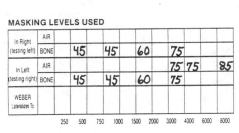

In Right (testing left)	AIR								
	BONE	45	45	60	75				
In Left (testing right)	AIR					75	75		85
	BONE	45	45	60	75				
WEBER Lateralizes To									
		250	500	750	1000	1500	2000	3000	4000	6000	8000

PURE-TONE AUDIOGRAM
FREQUENCY IN HERTZ (Hz)

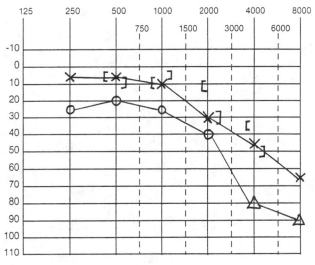

EVALUATION _____

_____

_____

_____

_____

_____

_____

_____

_____

_____

INTERPRETATION

RIGHT EAR: Mild, steeply sloping to severe, mixed hearing loss. Only fair word discrimination. Could not evaluate middle ear status with tympanometry due to the fluid in the ear canal.

LEFT EAR: Mild-to-moderate high frequency SN loss. Only fair speech discrimination. Normal middle ear function per tympanometry. No acoustic reflex AU.

PRESENTING INFORMATION

Pt. is a welder who sustained a burn in his left ear canal from welding material about 8 days ago. Several days later, he was injured in a motorcycle accident. He was not wearing a helmet. He presents with orthopedic injuries and road burns. There is dried blood in each ear canal. He complains of unsteadiness and a full feeling in the left ear, which began after the welding burn. He also reports a hx of exposure to high-level noise.

MIDDLE EAR MEASURES:		RIGHT	LEFT
	MEV:	1.0 ml	1.0 ml
	COMP:	.5 ml	.2 ml
	MEP:	-42 daPa	-140 daPa

Pt. Information:

M __X__ F _____ Age: __39__

PURE-TONE AUDIOGRAM
FREQUENCY IN HERTZ (Hz)

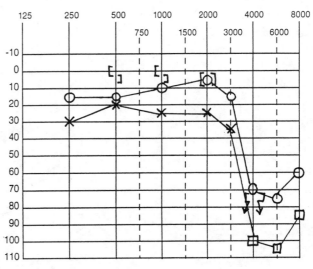

SPEECH AUDIOMETRY

	SRT		WORD RECOGNITION		
	dB	Mask	%	Mask	SL
RIGHT	10		92		30
LEFT	30		100	50	30
RIGHT					
LEFT					
BIN					

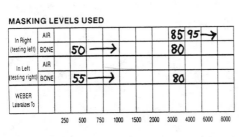

MASKING LEVELS USED

In Right (testing left)	AIR							85	95 →
	BONE	50 →					80		
In Left (testing right)	AIR								
	BONE	55 →					80		
WEBER Lateralizes To									

250 500 750 1000 1500 2000 3000 4000 6000 8000

EVALUATION _____

_____

_____

_____

_____

_____

_____

_____

INTERPRETATION

RIGHT EAR: Normal hearing through 3K Hz with a severe to profound high frequency SN loss. (Pt. has a significant hx of noise exposure.) Good word discrimination score. Normal middle ear compliance and pressure.

LEFT EAR: Mild conductive loss through 3000 Hz with severe-profound high frequency SN deficit. Weber refers to left. Excellent word discrimination score. The tympanogram reflects reduced middle ear compliance at negative pressure.

PRESENTING INFORMATION

Twenty-year-old male who sustained left TM trauma with a single tine of a comb shoved into his ear by his baby daughter. Bloody otorrhea. Left canal trauma. Question TM perforation.

MIDDLE EAR MEASURES:	RIGHT	LEFT
ECV:	.7 ml	.8 ml
COMP:	.4 ml	.8 ml
MEP:	-30 daPa	-130 daPa

Pt. Information:

M __X__ F ____ Age: __20__

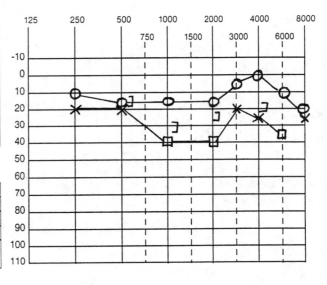

PURE-TONE AUDIOGRAM
FREQUENCY IN HERTZ (Hz)

SPEECH AUDIOMETRY					
	SRT		WORD RECOGNITION		
	dB	Mask	%	Mask	SL
RIGHT	5		100		30
LEFT	20		100	40	30
RIGHT					
LEFT					
BIN					

MASKING LEVELS USED

In Right (testing left)	AIR			55	55			50		
	BONE		50	60	60	50				
In Left (testing right)	AIR									
	BONE									
WEBER Lateralizes To										
		250	500	750	1000	1500	2000	3000	4000	6000	8000

EVALUATION _____

_____

_____

_____

_____

_____

_____

_____

_____

_____

INTERPRETATION

RIGHT EAR: Normal hearing sensitivity, speech discrimination, and normal middle ear compliance and pressure.

LEFT EAR: Mild, mixed hearing loss. Excellent speech discrimination score. Tympanometry was possible in spite of the condition of the ear canal. Results revealed normal middle ear compliance at negative pressure. The possibility of a TM perforation is not supported by these results.

PRESENTING INFORMATION

Fifty-year-old HIV positive male with over a 20-year-history of hearing loss and hearing aid use now presenting with gunshot wound (GSW) behind right ear. Wound has healed. Pt. complaining of bilateral ear pain and full feeling.

MIDDLE EAR MEASURES:		RIGHT	LEFT
	ECV:	.8 ml	1.0 ml
	COMP:	0 ml	.4 ml
	MEP:	Flat	- 15 daPa

Pt. Information:

M __X__ F _____ Age: _50_

SPEECH AUDIOMETRY

	SRT		WORD RECOGNITION		
	dB	Mask	%	Mask	SL
RIGHT	60		32	80	30
LEFT	50		80		30
RIGHT					
LEFT					
BIN					

MASKING LEVELS USED

In Right (testing left)	AIR							
	BONE							
In Left (testing right)	AIR	80	75		85		85	90 →
	BONE		80		90		95	95
WEBER Lateralizes To								

250 500 750 1000 1500 2000 3000 4000 6000 8000

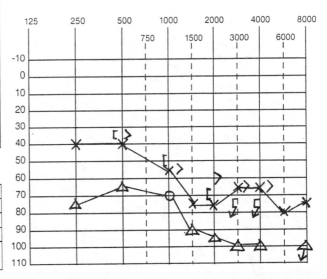

PURE-TONE AUDIOGRAM
FREQUENCY IN HERTZ (Hz)

EVALUATION _____

_____

_____

_____

_____

_____

_____

_____

_____

_____

INTERPRETATION

RIGHT EAR: Severe-profound mixed loss with a large SN component. Poor word discrimination score. Tympanometry reflects reduced physical volume and a noncompliant system which is consistent with the excessive cerumen obscuring the TM.

LEFT EAR: Mild-to-severe mixed loss with word discrimination ability. Tympanometry reveals normal middle ear compliance and pressure. There is excessive cerumen in the canal.

ENT NOTE

Asymmetric HL. Traumatic HL, AD. Cerumen cleared. TM's intact and compliant. Referred for new hearing aid.

PRESENTING INFORMATION

Hx of 37 years unprotected noise exposure in coal mines. Four-year hx of progressing hearing loss in left ear. Has had two ENT/audiology evaluations and was told that he was "uncooperative." No other dx was provided.

MIDDLE EAR MEASURES:	RIGHT	LEFT
ECV:	1.5 ml	1.9 ml
COMP:	1.8 ml	.4 ml
MEP:	- 25 daPa	-60 daPa

ACOUSTIC REFLEX ABSENT AU

Pt. Information:

M __X__ F _____ Age: **68**

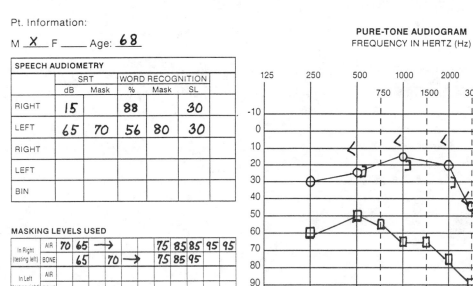

SPEECH AUDIOMETRY

	SRT		WORD RECOGNITION		
	dB	Mask	%	Mask	SL
RIGHT	15		88		30
LEFT	65	70	56	80	30
RIGHT					
LEFT					
BIN					

MASKING LEVELS USED

In Right (testing left)	AIR	70	65	→			75	85	85	95	95
	BONE		65		70	→		75	85	95	
In Left (testing right)	AIR										
	BONE										
WEBER Lateralizes To	L	✓	✓		✓						

250 500 750 1000 1500 2000 3000 4000 6000 8000

PURE-TONE AUDIOGRAM
FREQUENCY IN HERTZ (Hz)

EVALUATION _____

_____

_____

_____

_____

_____

_____

_____

_____

_____

INTERPRETATION

RIGHT EAR: Mild conductive loss through 2K Hz with a precipitous SNHL (mild to severe) in the high frequencies. The speech recognition score is consistent with mid-frequency pure tone AC thresholds. The discrimination score is fairly good. Middle ear compliance and pressure is WNL. The acoustic reflex is absent.

LEFT EAR: Moderate-to-moderately severe mixed loss with large conductive component through the low and mid frequencies. Severe-profound mixed loss above 1500 Hz. Very reduced word discrimination score. Weber refers to left. Although middle ear measurements are WNL, there is a significant reduction in compliance compared to his right ear. The acoustic reflex is absent.

RECOMMENDATION

Intertest and intratest agreement is good. He is advised to take these test results with him for a 3rd otologic opinion. He was provided with information re noise and hearing, and re hearing aids.

PRESENTING INFORMATION

Twenty one-year-old male with 5-month hx of left ear drainage. Recently treated for 10 days with amoxicillin for otitis media without improvement. Severe retraction of left TM (can see round window nitch). Large amount of yellow/white exudate. Right ear normal.

MIDDLE EAR MEASURES:

	RIGHT	LEFT
MEV:	1.4 ml	CNT
COMP:	.4 ml	
MEP:	- 30 daPa	

Pt. Information:

M _X_ F ____ Age: _21_

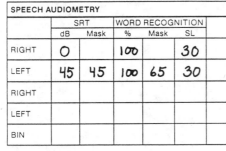

SPEECH AUDIOMETRY

	SRT		WORD RECOGNITION		
	dB	Mask	%	Mask	SL
RIGHT	0		100		30
LEFT	45	45	100	65	30
RIGHT					
LEFT					
BIN					

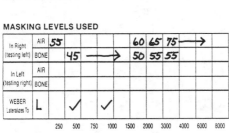

MASKING LEVELS USED

In Right (testing left)	AIR	55				60	65	75 →	
	BONE		45 →			50	55	55	
In Left (testing right)	AIR								
	BONE								
WEBER Lateralizes To	L	✓		✓					

250　500　750　1000　1500　2000　3000　4000　6000　8000

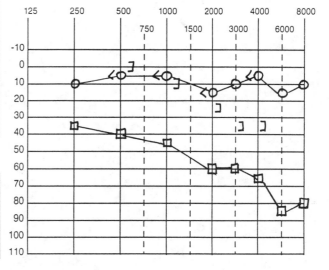

PURE-TONE AUDIOGRAM
FREQUENCY IN HERTZ (Hz)

EVALUATION _____

_____

_____

_____

_____

_____

_____

_____

_____

INTERPRETATION

RIGHT EAR: Hearing sensitivity and middle ear function are WNL. Word discrimination is excellent.

LEFT EAR: Mild-to-severe mixed (largely conductive) loss. Excellent discrimination score. CNT middle ear function due to exudate in canal.

OUTCOME

Dx: Cholesteatoma, left ear. Rec: Left tympanomastoidectomy.

PRESENTING INFORMATION

CC: Tinnitus AU.

Hx of right side head injury from a fall 4 years ago. Jaws "pop and lock" since. Hx of construction noise exposure.

Has been treated for SOM, AU.

MIDDLE EAR MEASURES:	RIGHT	LEFT
ECV:	1.0 ml	.9 ml
COMP:	.4 ml	.5 ml
MEP:	-30 daPa	-40 daPa

ACOUSTIC REFLEX PRESENT AU

Pt. Information:

M _X_ F _____ Age: _45_

SPEECH AUDIOMETRY

	SRT		WORD RECOGNITION		
	dB	Mask	%	Mask	SL
RIGHT	5		100		30
LEFT	20		100	45	30
RIGHT					
LEFT					
BIN					

MASKING LEVELS USED

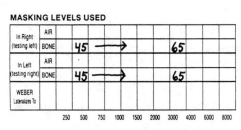

In Right (testing left)	AIR						
	BONE	45 →			65		
In Left (testing right)	AIR	.					
	BONE	45 →			65		
WEBER Lateralizes To							

250 500 750 1000 1500 2000 3000 4000 6000 8000

PURE-TONE AUDIOGRAM
FREQUENCY IN HERTZ (Hz)

EVALUATION _____

_____

_____

_____

_____

_____

_____

_____

_____

INTERPRETATION

NOTE: Narrow ear canals. Bilateral normal low and mid frequency thresholds with small air-bone gap. He has a mild-moderate, mixed, high frequency deficit. Both ears have excellent speech discrimination ability. Both ears have normal tympanograms.

IMPRESSION

The air-bone gap appears due to the narrowed ear canals.

ENT NOTE

TMJ dysfunction. Referred to oral surgery.

PRESENTING INFORMATION

Thirty nine-year-old with 15-year hx of sinusitis and asthma.
PE tube in left ear one year ago.
CC: Hearing loss.

MIDDLE EAR MEASURES:

	RIGHT	LEFT
ECV:	1.8 ml	2.2 ml
COMP:	2.3 ml	.25 ml
MEP:	-20 daPa	-90daP

Pt. Information:

M _____ F _X_ Age: _39_

SPEECH AUDIOMETRY

	SRT		WORD RECOGNITION		
	dB	Mask	%	Mask	SL
RIGHT	35		80		30
LEFT	35		92		30
RIGHT					
LEFT					
BIN					

MASKING LEVELS USED

In Right (testing left)	AIR								
	BONE	45	70	75	50				
In Left (testing right)	AIR								
	BONE	45	65	75	50				
WEBER Lateralizes To									

250 500 750 1000 1500 2000 3000 4000 6000 8000

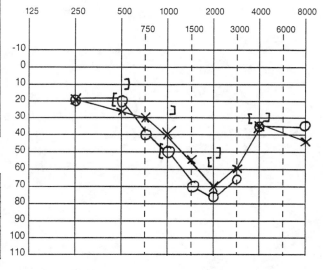

PURE-TONE AUDIOGRAM
FREQUENCY IN HERTZ (Hz)

EVALUATION _____

_____

_____

_____

_____

_____

_____

_____

_____

_____

_____

INTERPRETATION

Bilateral mild-to-severe mixed loss characterized by a large SN component and mid-frequency notch. Speech discrimination ability is only fair, right ear, and good, left ear.

Tympanometry reflects a hypercompliant right ME system (or TM) at normal pressure. The left tympanogram reveals increased physical volume and reduced compliance at mildly negative pressure which is not compatible with a patent PE tube.

RECOMMENDATION

Hearing aid evaluation when medical clearance can be provided for this pt.

PRESENTING INFORMATION

Referred by Oncology. Post-radiation evaluation (ca of tonsil). Pt. has significant hx of ear infections. Myringotomy with PE tube X3. Had left ear "reconstruction" surgery 3 years ago. Has PE tube in each ear at present.

MIDDLE EAR MEASURES:

	RIGHT	LEFT
MEV:	+6.0 ml	+6.0 ml

Pt. Information:

M __X__ F _____ Age: __46__

PURE-TONE AUDIOGRAM
FREQUENCY IN HERTZ (Hz)

SPEECH AUDIOMETRY

	SRT		WORD RECOGNITION		
	dB	Mask	%	Mask	SL
RIGHT	15		100		35
LEFT	45	40	80	50	30
RIGHT					
LEFT					
BIN					

MASKING LEVELS USED

In Right (testing left)	AIR	50 →		60 →			75	75
	BONE		60 →			65 →		
In Left (testing right)	AIR							
	BONE							
WEBER Lateralizes To								
		250	500	750	1000	1500	2000	3000	4000	6000	8000

EVALUATION

_____

_____

_____

_____

_____

_____

_____

_____

_____

_____

_____

_____

_____

_____

_____

INTERPRETATION

RIGHT EAR: Slight high frequency hearing loss. Excellent speech discrimination score.

LEFT EAR: Mild-to-profound mixed hearing loss with fairly good speech discrimination ability.

TYMPANOMETRY: Large physical volume AU (consistent with bilateral patent PE tubes).

PRESENTING INFORMATION

This man fell from 20-40 feet. He sustained severe head injuries including temporal bone fx. Required one month Rx in rehabilitative facility. Here to assess hearing status. Pt. is blind in left eye from previous MVA. ENT exam: TM's normal bilaterally. Dried blood in left ear canal.

MIDDLE EAR MEASURES:

	RIGHT	LEFT
ECV:	1.3 ml	.9 ml
COMP:	1.0 ml	.7 ml
MEP:	-20 daPa	-30 daPa

ACOUSTIC REFLEX PRESENT AD, ABSENT AS.

Pt. Information:

M __X__ F _____ Age: __41__

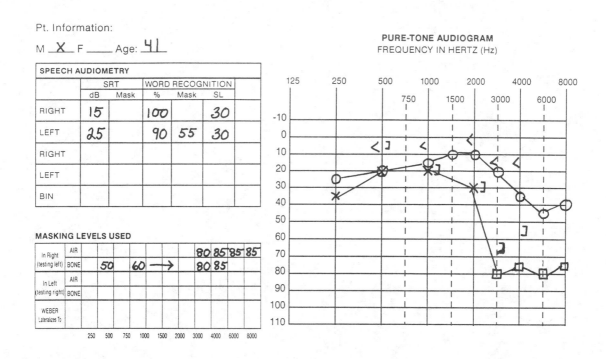

SPEECH AUDIOMETRY

	SRT		WORD RECOGNITION		
	dB	Mask	%	Mask	SL
RIGHT	15		100		30
LEFT	25		90	55	30
RIGHT					
LEFT					
BIN					

MASKING LEVELS USED

In Right (testing left)	AIR					80	85	85	85
	BONE	50	60	→		80	85		
In Left (testing right)	AIR								
	BONE								
WEBER Lateralizes To									

| | 250 | 500 | 750 | 1000 | 1500 | 2000 | 3000 | 4000 | 6000 | 8000 |

EVALUATION _____

_____

_____

_____

_____

_____

_____

_____

_____

INTERPRETATION

RIGHT EAR: Borderline normal to mild-moderate essentially conductive hearing loss. Normal tympanogram with acoustic reflex present. Normal hearing for speech and excellent speech discrimination ability.

LEFT EAR: Mild mixed loss through the low and mid frequencies with a severe, mixed high-frequency deficit. Normal tympanogram in spite of dried blood in ear canal. The acoustic reflex is absent.

RECOMMENDATION

Hearing retest following cleaning of ear canals.

PRESENTING INFORMATION

Pt. reports hearing loss present for 10-12 years. Wears 8-year-old hearing aid on left ear. Hx of Gentamycin Rx 20 years ago with no noticeable auditory sequela.

MIDDLE EAR MEASURES:

	RIGHT	LEFT
MEV:	1.3 ml	1.5 ml
COMP:	.4 ml	0 ml
MEP:	0 daPa	Flat

ACOUSTIC REFLEX PRESENT BELOW 2K Hz, AD

Pt. Information:

M _____ F __X__ Age: _56_

SPEECH AUDIOMETRY

	SRT		WORD RECOGNITION		
	dB	Mask	%	Mask	SL
RIGHT	20		100		30
LEFT	45		100	65	30
RIGHT					
LEFT					
BIN					

MASKING LEVELS USED

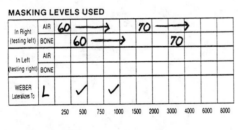

In Right (testing left)	AIR	60 →		70 →			
	BONE		60 →			70	
In Left (testing right)	AIR						
	BONE						
WEBER Lateralizes To	L	✓	✓				

250 500 750 1000 1500 2000 3000 4000 6000 8000

PURE-TONE AUDIOGRAM
FREQUENCY IN HERTZ (Hz)

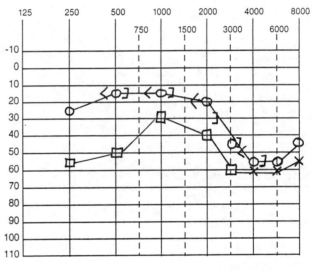

EVALUATION

_____

_____

_____

_____

_____

_____

_____

_____

_____

_____

INTERPRETATION

RIGHT EAR: Normal, or mildly depressed hearing 250 through 2K Hz with a moderate SN loss at the high frequencies. Excellent speech discrimination ability. Normal middle ear function per tympanometry. The acoustic reflex is present only below 2K Hz.

LEFT EAR: Mild-to-moderately severe mixed loss. Excellent discrimination score. The tympanogram is flat with normal physical volume. Weber refers to left.

ENT Dx

Left otosclerosis or other middle ear fixation problem. Cleared for binaural hearing aid use.

PRESENTING INFORMATION

Progressing hearing loss for many years. Here for evaluation today at family's insistence. She is very dependent on them, and they have great difficulty communicating with her. Ear canals are clear, and TM's appear normal.

MIDDLE EAR MEASURES:

	RIGHT	LEFT
ECV:	2.0 ml	1.5 ml
COMP:	1.0 ml	.7 ml
MEP:	-40 daPa	-70 daPa

Pt. Information:

M _____ F _X_ Age: _62_

SPEECH AUDIOMETRY

	SRT		WORD RECOGNITION		
	dB	Mask	%	Mask	SL
RIGHT	40		96		35
LEFT	80	60	100	80	25 (limits)
RIGHT					
LEFT					
BIN					

MASKING LEVELS USED

		250	500	750	1000	1500	2000	3000	4000	6000	8000
In Right (testing left)	AIR	85	85		80		85 →			90	90
	BONE		85	→			90	90	90		
In Left (testing right)	AIR										
	BONE										
WEBER Lateralizes To	L			✓		✓		✓			

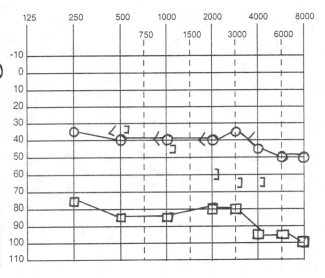

PURE-TONE AUDIOGRAM
FREQUENCY IN HERTZ (Hz)

EVALUATION

_____

_____

_____

_____

_____

_____

_____

_____

_____

_____

INTERPRETATION

RIGHT EAR: Mild-moderate SN hearing loss with very good speech discrimination ability. Middle ear compliance and pressure are WNL per tympanometry.

LEFT EAR: Severe mixed hearing loss. Weber supports the conductive component as does the excellent speech discrimination score. The tympanogram, however, shows normal compliance and pressure in the middle ear but does not rule out otosclerosis.

RECOMMENDATION

Referred for otologic evaluation. Amplification should be considered as soon as there is medical clearance for hearing aid use.

PRESENTING INFORMATION

Pt. complains of left ear hearing loss, otalgia, and occasional discharge in canal. He had chronic infections in this ear during childhood.

MIDDLE EAR MEASURES:

	RIGHT	LEFT
ECV:	1.4 ml	1.8 ml
COMP:	.6 ml	0 ml
MEP:	0 daPa	Flat

Pt. Information:

M __X__ F _____ Age: **22**

PURE-TONE AUDIOGRAM
FREQUENCY IN HERTZ (Hz)

SPEECH AUDIOMETRY

	SRT dB	SRT Mask	WORD RECOGNITION %	WORD RECOGNITION Mask	WORD RECOGNITION SL
RIGHT	O		100		30
LEFT	45	45	100	60	30
RIGHT					
LEFT					
BIN					

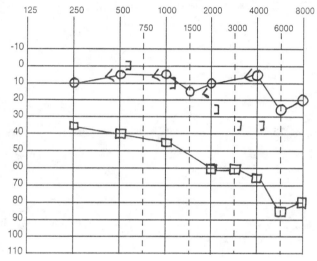

MASKING LEVELS USED

In Right (testing left)	AIR	55 →			60	60	65		75	75
In Right (testing left)	BONE		45 →		50	55	→			
In Left (testing right)	AIR									
In Left (testing right)	BONE									
WEBER Lateralizes To										

250 500 750 1000 1500 2000 3000 4000 6000 8000

EVALUATION

INTERPRETATION

RIGHT EAR: Hearing sensitivity and middle ear compliance and pressure are within normal limits. Word discrimination ability is excellent.

LEFT EAR: Mild to severe mixed (largely conductive) hearing loss. Excellent discrimination ability. Flat tympanogram at normal physical volume. Weber refers to left.

ENT IMPRESSIONS

Left Cholesteatoma. Scheduled for left tympanomastoidectomy.

PRESENTING INFORMATION

Fifty one-year-old woman with progressing hearing loss since age 28. She has had bilateral stapes mobilization surgery. She also has had 30 years of factory noise exposure.

MIDDLE EAR MEASURES:	RIGHT	LEFT
ECV:	1.7 ml	1.2 ml
COMP:	.5 ml	.8 ml
MEP:	0 daPa	0 daPa

NO ACOUSTIC REFLEX AD OR AS.

Pt. Information:

M _____ F _X_ Age: _51_

SPEECH AUDIOMETRY

	SRT		WORD RECOGNITION		
	dB	Mask	%	Mask	SL
RIGHT	55		88	75	30
LEFT	45		96	75	30
RIGHT					
LEFT					
BIN					

MASKING LEVELS USED

In Right (testing left)	AIR						
	BONE	75	80	85	90	90	
In Left (testing right)	AIR						
	BONE	80	80	80	85	90	
WEBER Lateralizes To		B	B				

250 500 750 1000 1500 2000 3000 4000 6000 8000

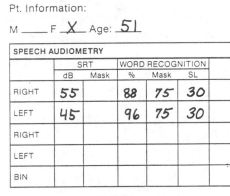

PURE-TONE AUDIOGRAM
FREQUENCY IN HERTZ (Hz)

EVALUATION _____

_____

_____

_____

_____

_____

_____

_____

_____

_____

INTERPRETATION

The auditory assessment reveals bilateral mild-moderate, low-frequency conductive hearing loss with a moderate-to-profound mixed loss from the mid through high frequencies. The speech discrimination score for the right ear is good and that for the left ear is excellent. Weber refers to both ears. Middle ear compliance and pressure are WNL per tympanometry. The acoustic reflex is absent AU.

RECOMMENDATION

Return to otologist for follow-up. (She has not had a medical evaluation in many years.) Replace 6-year-old hearing aids. Remove hearing aids when working near machinery.

PRESENTING INFORMATION

Malignant otitis externa AS. Brain scan revealed "an indolent infectious process in the left temporal region."

MIDDLE EAR MEASURES:

	RIGHT	LEFT
ECV:	2.0 ml	.5 ml
COMP:	.8 ml	0 ml
MEP:	- 35 daPa	Flat

Pt. Information:

M ____ F _X_ Age: _73_

SPEECH AUDIOMETRY

	SRT		WORD RECOGNITION		
	dB	Mask	%	Mask	SL
RIGHT	30		100		30
LEFT	40		100	60	30
RIGHT					
LEFT					
BIN					

MASKING LEVELS USED

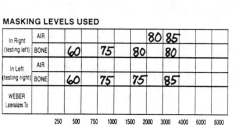

In Right (testing left) AIR						80	85			
In Right (testing left) BONE	60		75		80		80			
In Left (testing right) AIR										
In Left (testing right) BONE	60		75		75		85			
WEBER Lateralizes To										
	250	500	750	1000	1500	2000	3000	4000	6000	8000

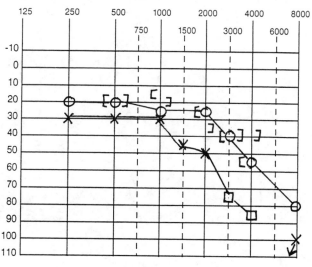

PURE-TONE AUDIOGRAM
FREQUENCY IN HERTZ (Hz)

EVALUATION _____

_____

_____

_____

_____

_____

_____

_____

_____

INTERPRETATION

RIGHT EAR: Borderline normal hearing thresholds 250 through 2K Hz with a precipitous high frequency SN HL. There is excellent speech discrimination ability and normal middle ear compliance and pressure.

LEFT EAR: Mild-moderate mixed low and mid frequency loss with a severe mixed loss above 3K Hz. Abnormal, noncompliant middle ear system function per tympanometry. The speech discrimination score is consistent with the nature of the loss.

PRESENTING INFORMATION

Pt. complains of right facial pain. There is a small superior TM perforation, right ear.

MIDDLE EAR MEASURES:	RIGHT	LEFT
ECV:	CNT	.7 ml
COMP:		.7 ml
MEP:		1.4 daPa

Pt. Information:

M _____ F _X_ Age: **55**

SPEECH AUDIOMETRY

	SRT		WORD RECOGNITION		
	dB	Mask	%	Mask	SL
RIGHT	70	55	92	75	30
LEFT	20		92		30
RIGHT					
LEFT					
BIN					

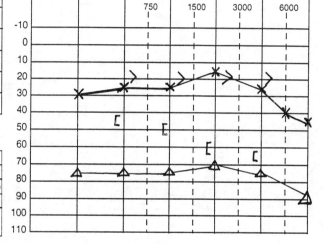

PURE-TONE AUDIOGRAM
FREQUENCY IN HERTZ (Hz)

MASKING LEVELS USED

In Right (testing left)	AIR								
	BONE								
In Left (testing right)	AIR	70	65	70	60	65	70	80	
	BONE		70	80	70	70			
WEBER Lateralizes To									
		250	500	750	1000	1500	2000	3000	4000	6000	8000

EVALUATION

_____

_____

_____

_____

_____

_____

_____

_____

_____

_____

_____

_____

_____

INTERPRETATION

RIGHT EAR: Severe mixed (essentially SN) hearing loss with good word discrimination score. Tympanometry could not be completed due to inability to seal the ear canal, supporting presence of a TM perforation.

LEFT EAR: Mild SN hearing loss with good word discrimination and normal tympanogram.

FOLLOW-UP

Pt. was referred by the ENT Clinic to oral surgery for evaluation of her facial pain.

PRESENTING INFORMATION

Pt. complains of pulsatile tinnitus and hearing loss, right ear. He experiences severe headaches, vertigo with vomiting, and loss of balance.

MIDDLE EAR MEASURES:	RIGHT	LEFT
ECV:	1.3 ml	1.1 ml
COMP:	1.9 ml	2.0 ml
MEP:	-40 daPa	-35 daPa

THE ACOUSTIC REFLEX IS PRESENT BUT REVERSED AD.
THE ACOUSTIC REFLEXES HAVE ELEVATED THRESHOLDS AND ARE REVERSED AS.
REFLEX AMPLITUDE IS MINIMAL AU.

Pt. Information:

M _X_ F _____ Age: _58_

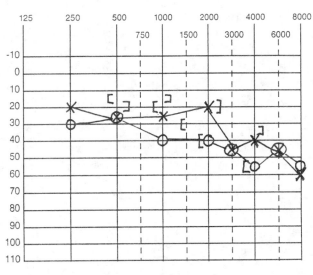

PURE-TONE AUDIOGRAM
FREQUENCY IN HERTZ (Hz)

SPEECH AUDIOMETRY

	SRT		WORD RECOGNITION		
	dB	Mask	%	Mask	SL
RIGHT	20		92		30
LEFT	20		92		30
RIGHT					
LEFT					
BIN					

MASKING LEVELS USED

In Right (testing left)	AIR							
	BONE	45	60	60	65			
In Left (testing right)	AIR							
	BONE	45	55	60	65			
WEBER Lateralizes To								
		250	500	750	1000	1500	2000	3000	4000	6000	8000

EVALUATION _____

_____
_____
_____
_____
_____
_____
_____
_____
_____

INTERPRETATION

The auditory assessment reveals bilateral mild-to-moderately severe mixed, essentially SN hearing loss. The right ear has poorer mid frequency sensitivity where there is an air-bone gap at 500 and 1K Hz. Speech discrimination ability is good AU. Tympanograms are normal.

The acoustic reflex has reduced amplitude in the right ear. There are reversed acoustic reflexes in each ear which would suggest either poor seals of the ear canals for these tests or the possibility of some middle ear fixation.

OUTCOME

The pt. was lost to follow-up.

PRESENTING INFORMATION

This pt. has very narrow, collapsed ear canals and a significant hearing loss. Her annual hearing tests for the past 3 years reveal stable bone conduction thresholds but an increase in the air conduction scores.

MIDDLE EAR MEASURES:	RIGHT	LEFT
ECV:	.4 ml	.6 ml
COMP:	.6 ml	.5 ml
MEP:	0 daPa	0 daPa

ACOUSTIC REFLEX IS PRESENT AU.

Pt. Information:

M ____ F _X_ Age: _75_

SPEECH AUDIOMETRY

	SRT		WORD RECOGNITION		
	dB	Mask	%	Mask	SL
RIGHT	65	70	40	85	30
LEFT	35		72		30
RIGHT					
LEFT					
BIN					

MASKING LEVELS USED

In Right (testing left)	AIR						
	BONE	85	80	95	100		
In Left (testing right)	AIR	75	70	80	85	100 →	
	BONE	75	75	85	90		
WEBER Lateralizes To							

250 500 750 1000 1500 2000 3000 4000 6000 8000

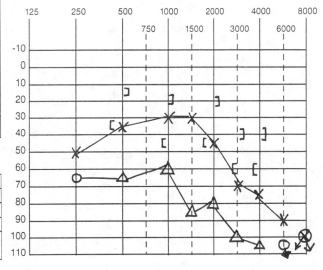

PURE-TONE AUDIOGRAM
FREQUENCY IN HERTZ (Hz)

EVALUATION _____

_____

_____

_____

_____

_____

_____

_____

_____

_____

INTERPRETATION

RIGHT EAR: Moderate, sloping to profound, mixed hearing loss. The speech discrimination score is very reduced.

LEFT EAR: Mild-moderate low and mid frequency mixed loss sloping to a severe high frequency deficit. Speech discrimination ability is fair.

TYMPANOMETRY: Small ear canal volume with normal middle ear pressure and compliance. The acoustic reflex is elicited at 500 and 1K Hz AU.

RECOMMENDATION

Assymetrical loss. R/O retrocochlear pathology. In terms of rehabilitation, binaural behind the ear hearing aids with sequentially enlarged earmolds may alter the ear canals as well as provide compensation for the hearing loss.

PRESENTING INFORMATION

Forty two-year-old woman status post head trauma with right CN VII paralysis. Also, complains of right ear hearing loss which may have improved during the past month. She has had facial nerve decompression surgery and has a gold weight in her right eyelid.

MIDDLE EAR MEASURES:

	RIGHT	LEFT
ECV:	CNT	1.5 ml
COMP:		.4 ml
MEP:		0 daPa

Pt. Information:

M _____ F _X_ Age: _42_

SPEECH AUDIOMETRY					
	SRT		WORD RECOGNITION		
	dB	Mask	%	Mask	SL
RIGHT	30	45	100	60	30
LEFT	10		100		30
RIGHT					
LEFT					
BIN					

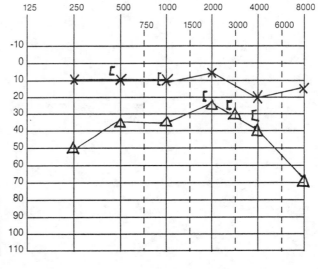

PURE-TONE AUDIOGRAM
FREQUENCY IN HERTZ (Hz)

MASKING LEVELS USED

In Right (testing left)	AIR							
	BONE							
In Left (testing right)	AIR	55 →		45 →			75	
	BONE	55 →						
WEBER Lateralizes To								
		250	500	750	1000 1500 2000	3000 4000	6000 8000	

EVALUATION _____

_____

_____

_____

_____

_____

_____

_____

_____

_____

_____

INTERPRETATION

RIGHT EAR: Mild, mixed hearing loss (except for a severe deficit at 8K Hz). Bone conduction thresholds have remained stable since her head injury and air conduction thresholds have improved. Word discrimination is excellent. Could not complete tympanometry due to medication in the ear canal.

LEFT EAR: Maintains normal hearing sensitivity and normal middle ear activity in this ear.

MIXED HL CASE #20

PRESENTING INFORMATION

Sixty four-year-old man with no prior history of ear problems now presents with a sudden hearing loss, AD, which occurred when he was coughing 7 days ago. He also is experiencing lightheadedness and loss of balance.

MIDDLE EAR MEASURES:

	RIGHT	LEFT
ECV:	1.5 ml	.9 ml
COMP:	.2 ml	.8 ml
MEP:	-150 daPa	-25 daPa

Pt. Information:

M X F ____ Age: 64

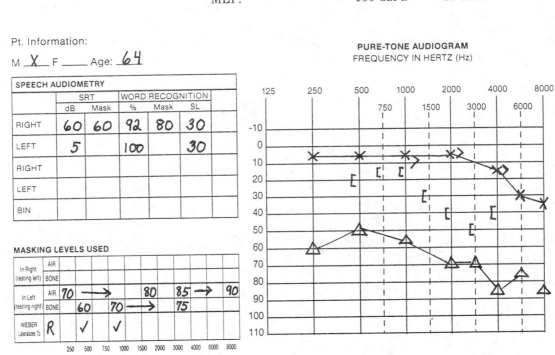

SPEECH AUDIOMETRY

	SRT		WORD RECOGNITION		
	dB	Mask	%	Mask	SL
RIGHT	60	60	92	80	30
LEFT	5		100		30
RIGHT					
LEFT					
BIN					

MASKING LEVELS USED

In Right (testing left)	AIR									
	BONE									
In Left (testing right)	AIR	70	→			80	85	→		90
	BONE	60	70	→		75				
WEBER Lateralizes To	R	✓		✓						

250 500 750 1000 1500 2000 3000 4000 6000 8000

EVALUATION

_____

_____
_____
_____
_____
_____
_____
_____
_____
_____
_____

INTERPRETATION

RIGHT EAR: Moderate-severe mixed loss. Speech discrimination ability remains good. The Weber refers to this ear. Tympanometry reveals a hypocompliant middle ear system and negative pressure. The fistula test was negative.

LEFT EAR: Normal hearing sensitivity 250 through 4K Hz with a mild, high-frequency SN deficit. Normal hearing for speech. Normal tympanogram.

PRESENTING INFORMATION

This pt. presents with a surgically enlarged left ear canal. She has a hx of exposure to loud music and motorcycles.

MIDDLE EAR MEASURES:		RIGHT	LEFT
	ECV:	.7 ml	CNT
	COMP:	.3 ml	
	MEP:	-75 daPa	

Pt. Information:

M _____ F **X** Age: **33**

SPEECH AUDIOMETRY

	SRT		WORD RECOGNITION		
	dB	Mask	%	Mask	SL
RIGHT	15		96		30
LEFT	25		96	50	30
RIGHT					
LEFT					
BIN					

MASKING LEVELS USED

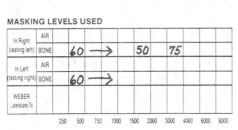

In Right (testing left)	AIR				
	BONE	60 →		50	75
In Left (testing right)	AIR				
	BONE	60 →			
WEBER Lateralizes To					

250 500 750 1000 1500 2000 3000 4000 6000 8000

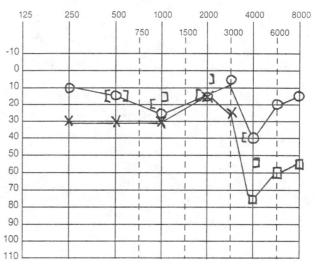

PURE-TONE AUDIOGRAM
FREQUENCY IN HERTZ (Hz)

EVALUATION

_____

_____

_____

_____

_____

_____

_____

_____

_____

_____

_____

INTERPRETATION

RIGHT EAR: Hearing thresholds are within normal limits with the exception of a mild SN deficit at 4000 Hz. The word discrimination score is excellent. The tympanogram reveals normal middle ear compliance at slight negative pressure.

LEFT EAR: There is a mild to moderately-severe mixed hearing loss. Speech discrimination ability is very good. Middle ear assessment with tympanometry could not be accomplished due to the altered shape and size of the ear canal.

PRESENTING INFORMATION

Pt. complains of right ear hearing loss and pulsatile tinnitus (synchronous with her pulse).

MIDDLE EAR MEASURES:	RIGHT	LEFT
ECV:	1.3 ml	1.5 ml
COMP:	.4 ml	.6 ml
MEP:	-180daP	0 daPa

ACOUSTIC REFLEX ABSENT IN RIGHT EAR, PRESENT IN LEFT EAR.
PULSATILE TRACINGS FOR RIGHT EAR TESTS.

Pt. Information:

M _____ F X Age: **68**

SPEECH AUDIOMETRY

	SRT		WORD RECOGNITION		
	dB	Mask	%	Mask	SL
RIGHT	30		96	55	30
LEFT	10		100		30
RIGHT					
LEFT					
BIN					

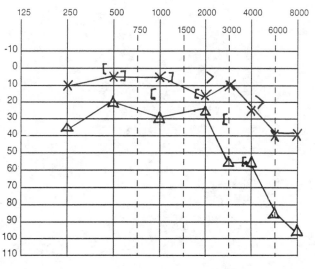

PURE-TONE AUDIOGRAM
FREQUENCY IN HERTZ (Hz)

MASKING LEVELS USED

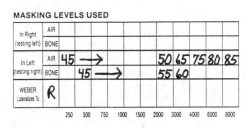

In Right (testing left)	AIR									
	BONE									
In Left (testing right)	AIR	45 →				50	65	75	80	85
	BONE	45 →				55	60			
WEBER Lateralizes To	R									

EVALUATION

_____

_____

_____

_____

_____

_____

_____

_____

_____

_____

INTERPRETATION

RIGHT EAR: Mild conductive hearing loss through 2000Hz with a precipitous mixed loss at higher frequencies. Hearing for speech is mildly impaired and speech discrimination ability remains very good. The tympanogram reveals significantly negative middle ear pressure but normal compliance. The acoustic reflex is absent in this ear. The test records a pulsatile component.

LEFT EAR: Normal hearing sensitivity with the exception of a mild high-frequency deficit above 4000 Hz. Excellent speech discrimination score. Normal tympanogram. The acoustic reflex is elicited at normal thresholds.

IMPRESSION

Asymmetric high frequency essentially SN hearing loss, AD, with a mild conductive loss for low and mid frequencies. Pulsatile middle ear. Absent acoustic reflex. R/O glomus tumor.

PRESENTING INFORMATION

CC: Right ear draining. This 44-year-old man had right tympanomastoid surgery with a middle ear prosthesis 6 years ago. He has not returned for evaluation in 5 years. He now has no right TM. The prosthesis is visible and in good condition.

MIDDLE EAR MEASURES:

	RIGHT	LEFT
ECV:	+5.0 ml	1.4 ml
COMP:	0	1.1 ml
MEP:	Flat	-48 daPa

Pt. Information:

M _X_ F ___ Age: **44**

SPEECH AUDIOMETRY

	SRT		WORD RECOGNITION		
	dB	Mask	%	Mask	SL
RIGHT	45	60	100	60	30
LEFT	10		100		30
RIGHT					
LEFT					
BIN					

MASKING LEVELS USED

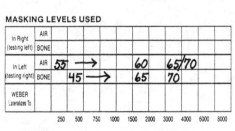

In Right (testing left)	AIR								
	BONE								
In Left (testing right)	AIR	55 →			60	65/70			
	BONE	45 →			65	70			
WEBER Lateralizes To									

| 250 | 500 | 750 | 1000 | 1500 | 2000 | 3000 | 4000 | 6000 | 8000 |

PURE-TONE AUDIOGRAM
FREQUENCY IN HERTZ (Hz)

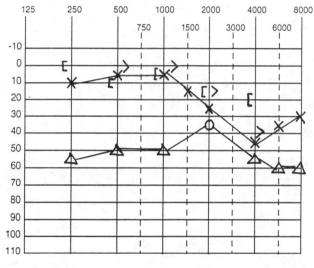

EVALUATION

_____

_____

_____

_____

_____

_____

_____

_____

_____

INTERPRETATION

RIGHT EAR: Moderately severe conductive hearing loss. Excellent speech discrimination score. Tympanometry measures a large physical volume indicative of TM perforation.

LEFT EAR: Normal hearing 250 through 1000 Hz sloping to a mild high-frequency SN hearing loss. The speech discrimination score is excellent. The tympanogram is WNL.

OUTCOME

Pt. was scheduled for a radical mastoidectomy.

PRESENTING INFORMATION

Seventeen-year-old trauma pt. with bilateral temporal bone fractures, right and left CN VII paralysis, right hemotympanum (intact TM), and left ear canal laceration and hemotympanum.

The pt. was tested at bedside in the intensive care unit. His condition required rapid assessment.

Pt. Information:

M _X_ F ____ Age: _17_

SPEECH AUDIOMETRY

	SRT dB	SRT Mask	WORD RECOGNITION %	WORD RECOGNITION Mask	WORD RECOGNITION SL
RIGHT	CNT				
LEFT	CNT				
RIGHT					
LEFT					
BIN					

MASKING LEVELS USED

In Right (testing left)	AIR									
	BONE									
In Left (testing right)	AIR									
	BONE									
WEBER Lateralizes To										

PURE-TONE AUDIOGRAM
FREQUENCY IN HERTZ (Hz)

EVALUATION

INTERPRETATION

Ambient room noise may have affected the validity of these test results.

RIGHT EAR: Mild low to mid frequency conductive loss with a moderate to profound high frequency, essentially SN deficit.

LEFT EAR: Mild, essentially conductive hearing loss.

PRESENTING INFORMATION

This pt. reported experiencing sharp pain and spontaneous bleeding from her right ear 7 days prior to this test.

MIDDLE EAR MEASURES:		RIGHT	LEFT
	ECV:	1.4 ml	.8ml
	COMP:	2.3 ml	1.6ml
	MEP:	0 daPa	0daP

THE ACOUSTIC REFLEX IS ELICITED AU.

Pt. Information:

M _____ F _X_ Age: _54_

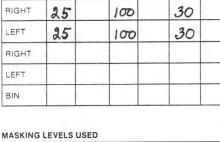

SPEECH AUDIOMETRY

	SRT		WORD RECOGNITION		
	dB	Mask	%	Mask	SL
RIGHT	25		100		30
LEFT	25		100		30
RIGHT					
LEFT					
BIN					

MASKING LEVELS USED

		250	500	750	1000	1500	2000	3000	4000	6000	8000
In Right (testing left)	AIR										
	BONE	60 →									
In Left (testing right)	AIR										
	BONE	60 →									
WEBER Lateralizes To											

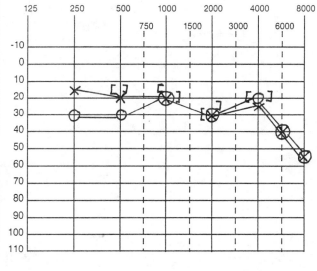

PURE-TONE AUDIOGRAM
FREQUENCY IN HERTZ (Hz)

EVALUATION _____

_____

_____

_____

_____

_____

_____

_____

_____

_____

_____

INTERPRETATION

Test results reveal bilateral borderline-normal hearing sensitivity except for a mild high-frequency deficit. There is a small air-bone gap at the low frequencies in the right ear. Hearing for speech is mildly impaired. Speech discrimination ability is excellent AU.

Both tympanograms reflect normal middle ear pressure. The right ear compliance is greater than that measured for the left ear. The acoustic reflex is present AU.

ENT DIAGNOSIS

Recovering bullous myringitis AD.

SECTION 4
NORMAL HEARING

PRESENTING INFORMATION

Pt. presents with complaint of severe right otalgia for past 20 hours. Hx of renal/pancreas transplant 4 months ago. He states that the ear pain has now moved to his face. He had a fever overnight. The right ear canal is clear. The TM is distended with blobs on TM and fluid in middle ear.

Arrangements were made for a sterile myringotomy and lab workup on the ME fluid samples. Following the aspiration of fluid, medication was placed in each canal, cotton blocks were inserted, and the pt. was referred for immediate auditory assessment.

Pt. Information:

M __X__ F _____ Age: __31__

SPEECH AUDIOMETRY

	SRT		WORD RECOGNITION		
	dB	Mask	%	Mask	SL
RIGHT	15		100		35
LEFT	10		100		35
RIGHT					
LEFT					
BIN					

MASKING LEVELS USED

In Right (testing left)	AIR									
	BONE	50 →								
In Left (testing right)	AIR									
	BONE	50 →								
WEBER Lateralizes To										

250 500 750 1000 1500 2000 3000 4000 6000 8000

PURE-TONE AUDIOGRAM
FREQUENCY IN HERTZ (Hz)

EVALUATION _____

_____

_____

_____

_____

_____

_____

_____

_____

_____

_____

INTERPRETATION

NOTE: Cotton present in both ear canals. Did not remove for test due to recent myringotomy and eardrops. Bilateral normal or borderline normal hearing sensitivity. No evidence of a significant conductive component, but it is noted that this test has followed the myringotomy. Hearing for speech is within normal limits, and discrimination scores are excellent. CNT middle ear function at this time.

ENT NOTE

Samples of middle ear material sent to lab. The differential diagnosis of bullous myringitis includes viral, mycoplasma, and tuberculous otitis.

NORMAL HEARING CASE #2

PRESENTING INFORMATION

Pt. presents on 4th day of right facial nerve paralysis.

MIDDLE EAR MEASURES:	RIGHT	LEFT
ECV:	2.0 ml	1.5 ml
COMP:	.4 ml	.4 ml
MEP:	0 daPa	0 daPa

ACOUSTIC REFLEX ABSENT, AD, AND PRESENT AT NORMAL THRESHOLDS AS.

Pt. Information:

M __X__ F _____ Age: _16_

SPEECH AUDIOMETRY

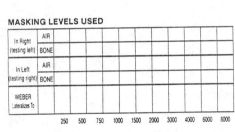

	SRT		WORD RECOGNITION		
	dB	Mask	%	Mask	SL
RIGHT	10		96		30
LEFT	10		100		30
RIGHT					
LEFT					
BIN					

MASKING LEVELS USED

		250	500	750	1000	1500	2000	3000	4000	6000	8000
In Right (testing left)	AIR										
	BONE										
In Left (testing right)	AIR										
	BONE										
WEBER Lateralizes To											

PURE-TONE AUDIOGRAM
FREQUENCY IN HERTZ (Hz)

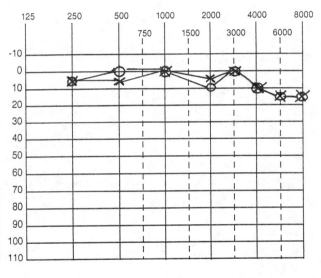

EVALUATION

_____

_____

_____

_____

_____

_____

_____

_____

_____

_____

INTERPRETATION

Auditory assessment reveals bilateral normal hearing sensitivity with normal hearing for speech and excellent word discrimination. Acoustic impedance measures reflect normal middle ear compliance and pressure AU. Acoustic reflex activity is normal in the left ear. The acoustic reflex is absent in the right ear.

These test results are consistent with the diagnosis of right Bell's palsy.

PRESENTING INFORMATION

The pt.'s cc is right ear tinnitus. It began several months ago and has increased in severity. She denies trauma, otalgia, dizziness, or loss of balance. She does have frequent headaches. She has a previous hx of factory noise exposure.

MIDDLE EAR MEASURES:	RIGHT	LEFT
ECV:	1.1 ml	1.1 ml
COMP:	1.4 ml	1.3 ml
MEP:	-130 dap	-50 daPa

THE ACOUSTIC REFLEX IS ABSENT IN THE RIGHT EAR WITH IPSILATERAL AND CONTRALATERAL STIMULATION.

LEFT EAR CONTRALATERAL REFLEXES ARE ELEVATED OR ABSENT.

LEFT IPSILATERAL REFLEXES ARE NORMAL.

Pt. Information:

M ____ F _X_ Age: **55**

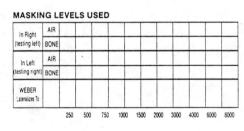

SPEECH AUDIOMETRY

	SRT		WORD RECOGNITION		
	dB	Mask	%	Mask	SL
RIGHT	**5**		**96**	**40**	**35**
LEFT	**5**		**96**	**40**	**35**
RIGHT					
LEFT					
BIN					

MASKING LEVELS USED

In Right (testing left)	AIR								
	BONE								
In Left (testing right)	AIR	.							
	BONE								
WEBER Lateralizes To									

250 500 750 1000 1500 2000 3000 4000 6000 8000

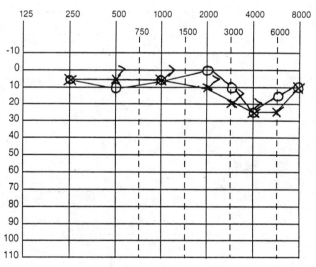

PURE-TONE AUDIOGRAM
FREQUENCY IN HERTZ (Hz)

EVALUATION _____

_____

_____

_____

_____

_____

_____

INTERPRETATION

Bilateral normal hearing sensitivity with the exception of a slight SN deficit around 4000 Hz. Detection of speech is normal with excellent word discrimination scores. The tympanograms reflect mildly negative middle ear pressure in the right ear and normal pressure in the left ear. Middle ear compliance is within normal limits AU. The ipsilateral acoustic reflex is absent in the right ear and present at normal thresholds in the left ear (without decay). With left ear stimulation, the contralateral reflex is absent. With right ear stimulation, the contralateral reflex is elevated or absent.

IMPRESSION

Tinnitus complaint AD. Abnormal acoustic reflex AD.
Recommending site of lesion evaluation to R/O right retrocochlear pathology.

PRESENTING INFORMATION

Thirty two-year-old woman complains of "dizziness" and unsteady gait for years. No vertigo. Her symptoms have worsened since sustaining injuries in a MVA (unrestrained driver) 11 months ago. No complaint of hearing loss or tinnitus. Rhomberg normal. Physical exam normal.

MIDDLE EAR MEASURES:	RIGHT	LEFT
ECV:	1.7 ml	1.3 ml
COMP:	.6 ml	.3 ml
MEP:	-30 daPa	-20 daPa

CONTRALATERAL ACOUSTIC REFLEX ACTIVITY IS NORMAL WITH LEFT EAR STIMULATION AND IS ABSENT WITH RIGHT EAR STIMULATION.

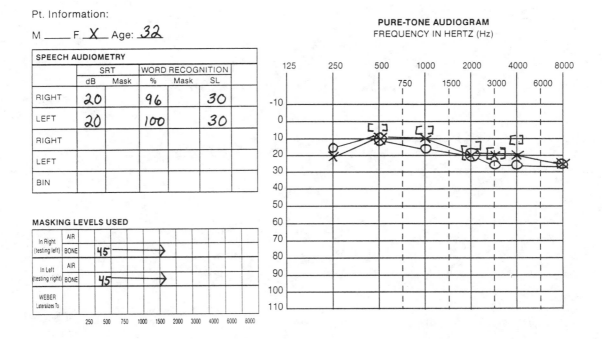

Pt. Information:

M _____ F _X_ Age: _32_

SPEECH AUDIOMETRY

	SRT		WORD RECOGNITION		
	dB	Mask	%	Mask	SL
RIGHT	20		96		30
LEFT	20		100		30
RIGHT					
LEFT					
BIN					

MASKING LEVELS USED

In Right (testing left)	AIR								
	BONE	45 →							
In Left (testing right)	AIR								
	BONE	45 →							
WEBER Lateralizes To									

250 500 750 1000 1500 2000 3000 6000 8000

PURE-TONE AUDIOGRAM
FREQUENCY IN HERTZ (Hz)

EVALUATION _____

_____

_____

_____

_____

_____

_____

INTERPRETATION

The auditory assessment reveals normal or borderline normal hearing sensitivity in each ear. Word discrimination scores are excellent. Both tympanograms are WNL in terms of middle ear compliance and pressure. The acoustic reflex is obtained in the left ear with right ear stimulation, but it is absent in the right with left ear stimulation.

RECOMMENDATION

Abnormal acoustic reflex activity. Special tests of auditory function are indicated.

OUTCOME

No further testing was ordered for this patient. The medical opinion was "dizziness most likely of CNS origin."

PRESENTING INFORMATION

Pt. has neurofibromatosis, frequent petit mal seizures, and is S/P VP shunt. She has a persistent complaint of awkward gait and frequent falling. The pt. had a seizure during pure tone audiometry that lasted about 5 minutes.

MIDDLE EAR MEASURES:	RIGHT	LEFT
ECV:	1.6 ml	2.5 ml
COMP:	.8 ml	.9 ml
MEP:	0 daPa	0 daPa

THE ACOUSTIC REFLEX IS ABSENT AU.

Pt. Information:

M _____ F _X_ Age: _38_

SPEECH AUDIOMETRY

	SRT		WORD RECOGNITION		
	dB	Mask	%	Mask	SL
RIGHT	10		96		30
LEFT	10		96		30
RIGHT					
LEFT					
BIN					

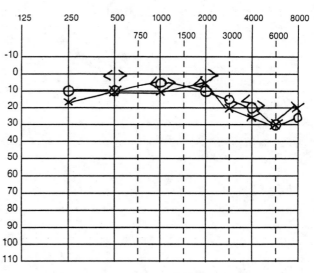

PURE-TONE AUDIOGRAM
FREQUENCY IN HERTZ (Hz)

MASKING LEVELS USED

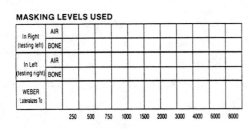

In Right (testing left)	AIR									
	BONE									
In Left (testing right)	AIR									
	BONE									
WEBER Lateralizes To										

250 500 750 1000 1500 2000 3000 4000 6000 8000

EVALUATION _____

_____

_____

_____

_____

_____

_____

_____

_____

INTERPRETATION

The auditory assessment revealed bilateral essentially normal hearing thresholds with the exception of a mild deficit at 6000 Hz. Acoustic impedance measures were normal for both ears, but the acoustic reflex is absent, bilaterally.

RECOMMENDATION

In view of the neurofibromatosis and the absence of the acoustic reflex in each ear, site of lesion tests are indicated to rule out retrocochlear pathology.

PRESENTING INFORMATION

Pt. with left VIIth nerve paralysis now complaining of severe left ear hyperacusis.

MIDDLE EAR MEASURES:

	RIGHT	LEFT
ECV:	1.2 ml	1.4 ml
COMP:	.6 ml	.6 ml
MEP:	0 daPa	0 daPa

THE ACOUSTIC REFLEX IS PRESENT IN THE RIGHT EAR AT NORMAL THRESHOLDS AND IS ABSENT IN THE LEFT EAR.

Pt. Information:

M _X_ F ____ Age: _58_

SPEECH AUDIOMETRY

	SRT dB	SRT Mask	WORD RECOGNITION %	Mask	SL
RIGHT	5		100		35
LEFT	5		100		35
RIGHT					
LEFT					
BIN					

MASKING LEVELS USED

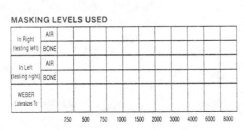

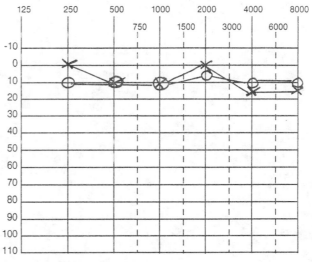

PURE-TONE AUDIOGRAM
FREQUENCY IN HERTZ (Hz)

EVALUATION

INTERPRETATION

Auditory assessment indicates bilateral normal hearing sensitivity with excellent speech discrimination ability. Acoustic impedance measures reveal normal middle ear function AU.

The acoustic reflex is present, probe right. The acoustic reflex is absent, probe left. This pattern is consistent with the VIIth nerve disorder.

PRESENTING INFORMATION:

Previously, this pt. complained of episodes of severe vertigo that lasted for days. She completed a trial with corticosteroids with no resolution of symptoms. An ENG was ordered, and the results were consistent with Menieres disease, left ear. A left endolymphatic shunt was performed 3 months ago.

MIDDLE EAR MEASURES:	RIGHT	LEFT
ECV:	1.5 ml	1.5 ml
COMP:	.6 ml	.5 ml
MEP:	0 daPa	-30daP

Pt. Information:

M _____ F _X_ Age: _29_

PURE-TONE AUDIOGRAM
FREQUENCY IN HERTZ (Hz)

SPEECH AUDIOMETRY

	SRT		WORD RECOGNITION		
	dB	Mask	%	Mask	SL
RIGHT	5		100		30
LEFT	10		100		30
RIGHT					
LEFT					
BIN					

MASKING LEVELS USED

In Right (testing left)	AIR									
	BONE									
In Left (testing right)	AIR									
	BONE									
WEBER Lateralizes To										
		250	500	750	1000	1500	2000	3000	4000	6000	8000

EVALUATION _____

_____

_____

_____

_____

_____

_____

_____

_____

_____

_____

INTERPRETATION

Postoperative test (left endolymphatic shunt). Test results reveal bilateral normal hearing sensitivity, excellent word discrimination, and normal middle ear function.

OUTCOME

The pt. had experienced no reoccurrence of vertigo at the time of this evaluation.

PRESENTING INFORMATION:

Pt.'s cc is of frequent, brief episodes of vertigo. He is HIV positive and has had several AIDS-related illnesses.

MIDDLE EAR MEASURES:	RIGHT	LEFT
ECV:	1.5 ml	CNT - Debris
COMP:	1.2 ml	
MEP:	0 daPa	

THE ACOUSTIC REFLEX IS PRESENT WITH RIGHT IPSILATERAL STIMULATION. THE LEFT EAR CANAL IS OBSTRUCTED.

Pt. Information:

M __X__ F _____ Age: _32_

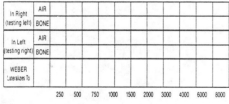

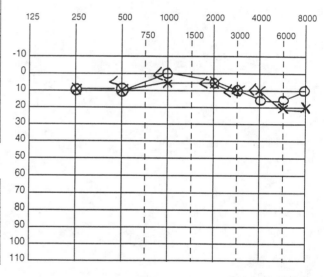

SPEECH AUDIOMETRY

	SRT dB	SRT Mask	WORD RECOGNITION %	WORD RECOGNITION Mask	WORD RECOGNITION SL
RIGHT	5		100		35
LEFT	5		100		35
RIGHT					
LEFT					
BIN					

MASKING LEVELS USED

In Right (testing left)	AIR									
	BONE									
In Left (testing right)	AIR									
	BONE									
WEBER Lateralizes To										
		250	500	750	1000	1500	2000	3000	4000	6000	8000

EVALUATION _____

_____

_____

_____

_____

_____

_____

_____

_____

INTERPRETATION

Bilateral normal hearing sensitivity. Bilateral excellent word discrimination ability. Normal right tympanogram; acoustic reflex thresholds are WNL. Could not seal the left canal for test. Debris blocks probe.

OUTCOME

Normal Auditory Brainstem Response test results.

PRESENTING INFORMATION

Pt. was struck on the right ear 3 weeks ago and sustained an anterior/inferior perforation of the TM. At this follow up, she complains of "fuzzy" hearing in that ear.

MIDDLE EAR MEASURES:		RIGHT	LEFT
	ECV:	4.9 ml	1.1 ml
	COMP:		2.7 ml
	MEP:	Flat	-25 daPa

Pt. Information:

M _____ F __X__ Age: _24_

SPEECH AUDIOMETRY

	SRT		WORD RECOGNITION		
	dB	Mask	%	Mask	SL
RIGHT	10		100		35
LEFT	5		100		35
RIGHT					
LEFT					
BIN					

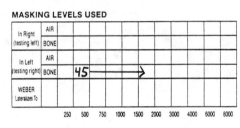

MASKING LEVELS USED

In Right (testing left)	AIR									
	BONE									
In Left (testing right)	AIR									
	BONE	45 ⟶								
WEBER Lateralizes To										

250 500 750 1000 1500 2000 3000 4000 6000 8000

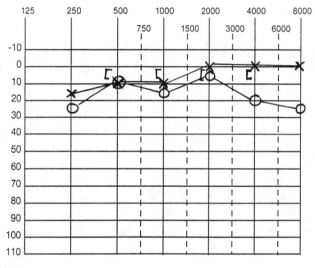

PURE-TONE AUDIOGRAM
FREQUENCY IN HERTZ (Hz)

EVALUATION

_____

_____

_____

_____

_____

_____

_____

_____

_____

_____

_____

INTERPRETATION

Hearing thresholds are essentially within normal limits with the exception of a mild deficit above 4000 Hz in the right ear. Speech reception thresholds are normal, and speech discrimination scores are excellent AU.

TYMPANOMETRY: Large physical volume AD, TM perforation. Hypercompliant system at normal pressure AS.

PRESENTING INFORMATION

Pt. complaining of dizziness since recovering from carbon monoxide poisoning with subsequent hyperbaric oxygen treatment last week. There is no complaint of hearing loss, tinnitus, or other neurologic difficulty.

MIDDLE EAR MEASURES:

	RIGHT	LEFT
ECV:	2.2 ml	1.3 ml
COMP:	1.0 ml	1.0 ml
MEP:	-90 daPa	-40 daPa

Pt. Information:

M __X__ F _____ Age: __57__

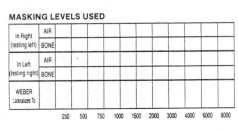

SPEECH AUDIOMETRY

	SRT		WORD RECOGNITION		
	dB	Mask	%	Mask	SL
RIGHT	O		100		30
LEFT	O		100		30
RIGHT					
LEFT					
BIN					

MASKING LEVELS USED

In Right (testing left)	AIR									
	BONE									
In Left (testing right)	AIR									
	BONE									
WEBER Lateralizes To										
		250	500	750	1000	1500	2000	3000	4000	6000	8000

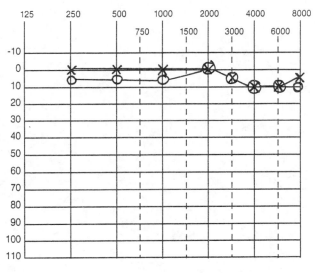

PURE-TONE AUDIOGRAM
FREQUENCY IN HERTZ (Hz)

EVALUATION _____

_____

_____

_____

_____

_____

_____

_____

_____

INTERPRETATION

The auditory assessment reveals bilateral normal hearing sensitivity with excellent speech discrimination ability AU. Middle ear measures reflect mildly negative middle ear pressure - greater in the right ear. Middle ear compliance is normal AU.

OUTCOME

"No apparent middle or inner ear damage." No treatment required. The patient reported that his dog appears to be deaf following the carbon monoxide exposure.

SECTION 5

NONORGANIC HEARING LOSS

PRESENTING INFORMATION

This woman is currently receiving medical and psychiatric treatment for an eating disorder. She has been referred for an assessment of her ears and hearing because she has recently claimed to be unable to hear her therapist. The ENT exam is WNL. During the auditory assessment, she had a flat affect and never made eye contact with the audiologist.

MIDDLE EAR MEASURES:		RIGHT	LEFT
	ECV:	1.9 ml	1.4 ml
	COMP:	.4 ml	1.1 ml
	MEP:	-30 daPa	-50 daPa

ACOUSTIC REFLEX PRESENT AT 1K Hz AND 2K Hz IN EACH EAR WITH 100 dB SCREENING.

Pt. Information:

M _____ F _X_ Age: _42_

SPEECH AUDIOMETRY

	SRT		WORD RECOGNITION		
	dB	Mask	%	Mask	SL
RIGHT	15		100		30
LEFT	45	50	100	60	30
RIGHT					
LEFT	35				
BIN					

MASKING LEVELS USED

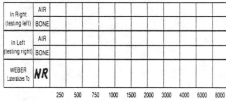

In Right (testing left)	AIR									
	BONE									
In Left (testing right)	AIR									
	BONE									
WEBER Lateralizes To	NR									

250 500 750 1000 1500 2000 3000 4000 6000 8000

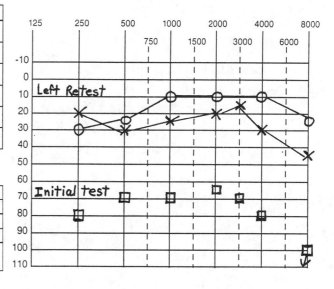

PURE-TONE AUDIOGRAM
FREQUENCY IN HERTZ (Hz)

Left Retest

Initial test

EVALUATION _____

_____

_____

_____

_____

_____

_____

_____

INTERPRETATION

The pt.'s initial left ear test results revealed a large discrepancy between her SRT and pure tone thresholds. Further testing led to a marked improvement in the pure tone thresholds (to borderline normal) and a 10 dB improvement in the SRT. There continues to be an unacceptable discrepancy between these two tests, however. Her tympanograms reveal normal middle ear function, and the acoustic reflex is present AU. Right ear test results were consistent and normal.

IMPRESSION

Nonorganic overlay, left ear test.

RECOMMENDATION

Reevaluate hearing status in one month.

OUTCOME

Two months following this exam, she was retested with no difficulty, and all hearing test results were normal.

PRESENTING INFORMATION

Pt. with rheumatoid arthritis and chronic otitis media is now seeking disability benefits. He did not respond when his name was called in the waiting area, and he cupped his ears in an exaggerated manner during his interview.

MIDDLE EAR MEASURES:		RIGHT	LEFT
	ECV:	2.6 ml	1.4 ml
	COMP:	1.8 ml	.4 ml
	MEP:	-90 daPa	-200 daPa

Pt. Information:

M **X** F _____ Age: **56**

SPEECH AUDIOMETRY

	SRT		WORD RECOGNITION		
	dB	Mask	%	Mask	SL
RIGHT	70	70	96	80	30
LEFT	25		100		30
RIGHT	35		100		30
LEFT	25		96		30
BIN					

MASKING LEVELS USED

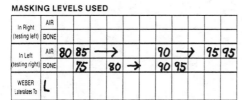

		250	500	750	1000	1500	2000	3000	4000	6000	8000
In Right (testing left)	AIR										
	BONE										
In Left (testing right)	AIR	80	85	→			90	→		95	95
	BONE		75		80	→		90	95		
WEBER Lateralizes To	L										

PURE-TONE AUDIOGRAM
FREQUENCY IN HERTZ (Hz)

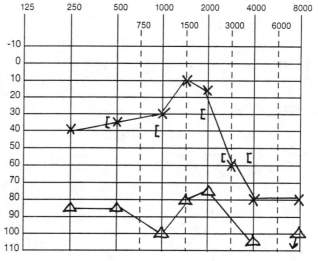

EVALUATION _____

_____

_____

_____

_____

_____

_____

_____

_____

_____

INTERPRETATION

RIGHT EAR: Test results of poor reliability. Severe-profound mixed hearing loss with large air-bone gap. He gave only half word responses to the speech recognition test and that threshold measure does not agree with pure tone thresholds.

LEFT EAR: Masking delimma: Could not adequately mask right ear for left ear B/C test. The Weber referred to left in spite of the audiometric evidence of a large right ear conductive component. Mild, presumably conductive, loss at low frequencies; steep mixed loss (essentially SN) above 2K Hz.

TYMPANOMETRY: The right tympanogram reflects a large physical volume, but compliance is WNL at mildly negative pressure. The left ear test reveals normal compliance at negative ME pressure.

OUTCOME

Hearing retest 7 months later revealed bilateral symmetrical borderline normal hearing through 2000 Hz with a severe high frequency SN deficit.

PRESENTING INFORMATION

Pt. referred from the ER and psychiatry. She states that she has just been raped by her taxi driver, and in trying to escape, she struck her left ear on the cab door and cannot hear from that ear. During testing, the pt. appeared to not be aware of where she was or what she was doing. She would remove the earphones frequently. Twice she stood up and rapidly began to undress.

MIDDLE EAR MEASURES: NORMAL ME VOLUME AND COMPLIANCE AT SLIGHTLY NEGATIVE PRESSURE AU. ACOUSTIC REFLEX PRESENT AU.

Pt. Information:

M _____ F _X_ Age: _28_

SPEECH AUDIOMETRY

	SRT		WORD RECOGNITION		
	dB	Mask	%	Mask	SL
RIGHT	15		NR		
LEFT	NR				
RIGHT					
LEFT	15		NR		
BIN					

MASKING LEVELS USED

In Right (testing left)	AIR									
	BONE									
In Left (testing right)	AIR									
	BONE									
WEBER Lateralizes To										

250　500　750　1000　1500　2000　3000　4000　6000　8000

PURE-TONE AUDIOGRAM
FREQUENCY IN HERTZ (Hz)

EVALUATION

_____

_____

_____

_____

_____

_____

_____

_____

_____

INTERPRETATION

The auditory assessment was difficult to complete because this patient seemed only vaguely aware of her surroundings and the tasks involved. She repeatedly removed the earphones and required frequent reinstruction.

The test results reveal bilateral normal hearing sensitivity in the speech range. Initially, she would not respond to left ear speech test presentations but later testing revealed that her word recognition is WNL in each ear. Her replies during word discrimination tests consisted of words that were related to the test items. No score for that test can be reported. Middle ear measures are within normal limits AU, and the acoustic reflex is present AU.

IMPRESSION

Normal, symmetrical hearing sensitivity in the speech frequencies.

PRESENTING INFORMATION

This pt. has been followed for bilateral moderate to severe high frequency SN loss since childhood. She had worn a high-frequency emphasis aid on the right ear since age 9. She has mild CP and is mildly retarded. Within the past year, her right ear was explored for a fistula, and postoperatively, there was a profound SN loss in this ear. Now, her family states that she is not responding to any sound and appears to have suddenly lost all hearing in the left ear.

We noted that she did not respond to anything that her mother said, but the pt. was able to converse freely with the audiologist. Her ABR test could not be interpreted due to her extraneous movements, and a sedated test has been recommended. An earlier ABR confirmed the profound loss AD.

MIDDLE EAR MEASURES: NORMAL COMPLIANCE AND PRESSURE.
IPSILATERAL ACOUSTIC REFLEXES: 100 @ 500Hz   90 @ 1K Hz   95 @ 2K Hz

Pt. Information:

M _____ F _X_ Age: _20_

SPEECH AUDIOMETRY

	SRT		WORD RECOGNITION			
	dB	Mask	%	Mask	SL	
RIGHT	NR					
LEFT	60		60		20	
RIGHT						
LEFT	75		72		15	MCL
BIN						

MASKING LEVELS USED

In Right (testing left)	AIR										
	BONE										
In Left (testing right)	AIR										
	BONE										
WEBER Lateralizes To											
		250	500	750	1000	1500	2000	3000	4000	6000	8000

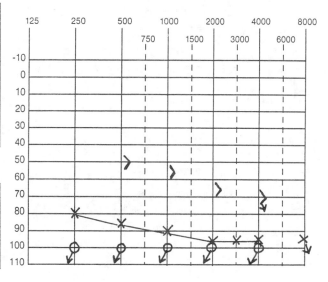

PURE-TONE AUDIOGRAM
FREQUENCY IN HERTZ (Hz)

EVALUATION _____

_____

_____

_____

_____

_____

INTERPRETATION

There is considerable evidence of nonorganic overlay on these left ear test results. There is poor inter and intra test reliability. Note that acoustic reflexes are present near or better than admitted pure tone thresholds. Her speech recognition thresholds are better than her A/C thresholds. During word discrimination tests, she repeats every other word. When the NR words are presented in list form, she again follows that pattern. Her organic level of hearing has not been identified on these tests.

OUTCOME

The otologist (with careful consideration) advised the pt.'s mother of the unusual test behavior and recommended psychiatric evaluation.

An ABR was attempted, but she would not sit quietly, and the test could not be completed. Retest with sedation is recommended.

PRESENTING INFORMATION

Pt. complains of blocked feeling in her right ear and inability to hear with that ear on the telephone. The otologic report states that she has acute otitis media with TM retraction, AD, and normal ear conditions AS. During the hearing evaluation, the pt. never responded to right ear tests. The Pure Tone Stenger Test was positive with right interference of 45 dB @ 500 Hz and 65 dB @ 1K Hz.

MIDDLE EAR MEASURES:

	RIGHT	LEFT
ECV:	3.0 ml	1.0 ml
COMP:	.2 ml	.4 ml
MEP:	Flat	-30 daPa

Pt. Information:

M _____ F _X_ Age: _32_

SPEECH AUDIOMETRY

	SRT dB	SRT Mask	WORD RECOGNITION %	WORD RECOGNITION Mask	WORD RECOGNITION SL
RIGHT	NR				
LEFT	15		100		30
RIGHT					
LEFT					
BIN					

MASKING LEVELS USED

		250	500	750	1000	1500	2000	3000	4000	6000	8000
In Right (testing left)	AIR										
	BONE										
In Left (testing right)	AIR										
	BONE										
WEBER Lateralizes To											

PURE-TONE AUDIOGRAM
FREQUENCY IN HERTZ (Hz)

EVALUATION

_____
_____
_____
_____
_____
_____
_____
_____
_____

INTERPRETATION

Auditory assessment revealed exaggerations of test thresholds. She gave no response to any right ear test, and the hearing status in that ear has not been established. The Pure Tone Stenger Test (which was positive) suggests a moderate to severe loss in this ear. The left ear (after some initial exaggeration of thresholds) appears to have normal hearing sensitivity.

The left tympanogram is normal. The right tympanogram reveals a hypocompliant system with a large physical volume.

RECOMMENDATION

Reevaluate hearing status in (at least) 3 weeks.

OUTCOME

The pt. continued to exaggerate her hearing thresholds on retest.

SECTION 6
PRACTICE AUDIOGRAMS

PRACTICE AUDIOGRAMS

The following are brief summaries of the presenting information that accompany the 15 practice tests.

PRACTICE CASE #1

Pt. has a large aneurysm originating from the left carotid siphon at the level of the posterior communicating artery.

MIDDLE EAR VOLUME, PRESSURE, AND COMPLIANCE ARE WNL AU.

Pt. Information:

M _____ F _X_ Age: _51_

SPEECH AUDIOMETRY

	SRT		WORD RECOGNITION		
	dB	Mask	%	Mask	SL
RIGHT	15		100		30
LEFT	25	40	84	50	30
RIGHT					
LEFT					
BIN					

MASKING LEVELS USED

In Right (testing left)	AIR						45	50	50	60	70	70
	BONE		50		50	55	60	→		70	
In Left (testing right)	AIR										
	BONE										
WEBER Lateralizes To	L	✓									

250 500 750 1000 1500 2000 3000 4000 6000 8000

PURE-TONE AUDIOGRAM
FREQUENCY IN HERTZ (Hz)

EVALUATION
_____
_____
_____
_____
_____
_____
_____
_____
_____
_____
_____

PRACTICE CASE #2

Hx of chronic ME disease AS. Preoperative test. Left mastoid resection planned.

MIDDLE EAR MEASURES:

	RIGHT	LEFT
ECV:	1.9 ml	4.0 ml
COMP:	.8 ml	0 ml
MEP:	0 daPa	Flat

Pt. Information:

M _____ F **X** Age: **66**

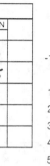

SPEECH AUDIOMETRY

	SRT		WORD RECOGNITION		
	dB	Mask	%	Mask	SL
RIGHT	15		100		30
LEFT	70	70	88	75	25
RIGHT					
LEFT					
BIN					

PURE-TONE AUDIOGRAM
FREQUENCY IN HERTZ (Hz)

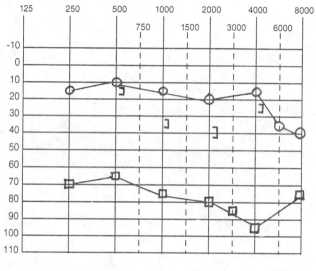

MASKING LEVELS USED

In Right (testing left)	AIR	80	80		85		90	100 →
	BONE		60		65	→		
In Left (testing right)	AIR							
	BONE							
WEBER Lateralizes To	L	✓		✓				

250 500 750 1000 1500 2000 3000 4000 6000 8000

EVALUATION _____

_____

_____

_____

_____

_____

_____

_____

_____

_____

_____

_____

_____

_____

PRACTICE CASE #3

Pt. states that he fell off his couch last night and is experiencing severe pain and some hearing loss in the left ear. Denies hx of ear or hearing problem. Otologic exam reveals a traumatic hemotympanum, AS, and a left lower neck mass. Will have CT.

MIDDLE EAR MEASURES:

	RIGHT	LEFT
ECV:	1.3 ml	.9 ml
COMP:	.5 ml	0 ml
MEP:	-20 daPa	Flat

Pt. Information:

M _X_ F _____ Age: _34_

SPEECH AUDIOMETRY

	SRT		WORD RECOGNITION		
	dB	Mask	%	Mask	SL
RIGHT	30		100		30
LEFT	40		100		30
RIGHT					
LEFT					
BIN					

MASKING LEVELS USED

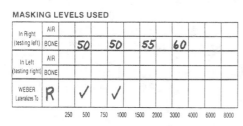

In Right (testing left)	AIR										
	BONE	50	50	55	60						
In Left (testing right)	AIR										
	BONE										
WEBER Lateralizes To	R	✓	✓								

250 500 750 1000 1500 2000 3000 4000 6000 8000

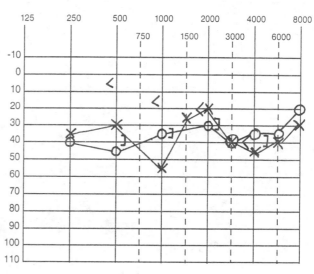

PURE-TONE AUDIOGRAM
FREQUENCY IN HERTZ (Hz)

EVALUATION _____

_____

_____

_____

_____

_____

_____

_____

_____

_____

_____

_____

PRACTICE CASE #4

Face crushed in MVA. Required left orbital decompression and tracheostomy. Hearing status is questioned. Pt. in distress and rapid testing at bedside was required.

MIDDLE EAR MEASURES:

		RIGHT	LEFT
ECV:		1.2 ml	1.1 ml
COMP:		4.2 ml	0 ml
MEP:		0 daPa	Flat

Pt. Information:

M ___ F _X_ Age: _26_

SPEECH AUDIOMETRY

	SRT dB	SRT Mask	WORD RECOGNITION %	WORD RECOGNITION Mask	WORD RECOGNITION SL
RIGHT	DNT				
LEFT	DNT				
RIGHT					
LEFT					
BIN					

MASKING LEVELS USED

		250	500	750	1000	1500	2000	3000	4000	6000	8000
In Right (testing left)	AIR	45	50		45						60
In Right (testing left)	BONE	50 →									
In Left (testing right)	AIR										
In Left (testing right)	BONE	60 →									
WEBER Lateralizes To											

PURE-TONE AUDIOGRAM
FREQUENCY IN HERTZ (Hz)

EVALUATION

_____

_____

_____

_____

_____

_____

_____

_____

_____

_____

_____

_____

_____

PRACTICE CASE #5

Pt. has AIDS. Confined to wheelchair but appears WDWN. He reports having rapidly progressing hearing loss for 5 months.

MIDDLE EAR MEASURES:

	RIGHT	LEFT
ECV:	1.6 ml	1.5 ml
COMP:	1.3 ml	.8 ml
MEP:	-25 daPa	-20 daPa

Pt. Information:

M _X_ F _____ Age: _35_

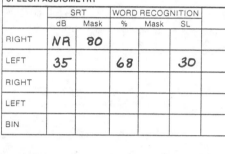

SPEECH AUDIOMETRY

	SRT		WORD RECOGNITION		
	dB	Mask	%	Mask	SL
RIGHT	NR	80			
LEFT	35		68		30
RIGHT					
LEFT					
BIN					

MASKING LEVELS USED

In Right (testing left)	AIR							
	BONE							
In Left (testing right)	AIR	90	90		85		80		90
	BONE		90		85		85		90
WEBER Lateralizes To	L		✓		✓			

250 500 750 1000 1500 2000 3000 4000 6000 8000

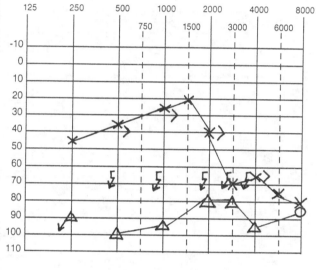

PURE-TONE AUDIOGRAM
FREQUENCY IN HERTZ (Hz)

EVALUATION _____

_____

_____

_____

_____

_____

_____

_____

_____

_____

_____

_____

_____

PRACTICE CASE #6

Hx of chronic otitis media. Now has left attic retraction. Cholesteatoma. Surgery scheduled.

MIDDLE EAR MEASURES:

	RIGHT	LEFT
ECV:	1.6 ml	1.4 ml
COMP:	2.0 ml	.7 ml
MEP:	-50 daPa	-260 daPa

Pt. Information:

M __X__ F _____ Age: __47__

SPEECH AUDIOMETRY

	SRT		WORD RECOGNITION		
	dB	Mask	%	Mask	SL
RIGHT	5		100		30
LEFT	15		100		30
RIGHT					
LEFT					
BIN					

MASKING LEVELS USED

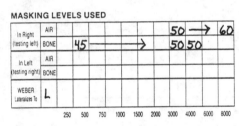

In Right (testing left)	AIR						50 → 60
	BONE	45 →					50 50
In Left (testing right)	AIR						
	BONE						
WEBER Lateralizes To	L						

250 500 750 1000 1500 2000 3000 4000 6000 8000

PURE-TONE AUDIOGRAM
FREQUENCY IN HERTZ (Hz)

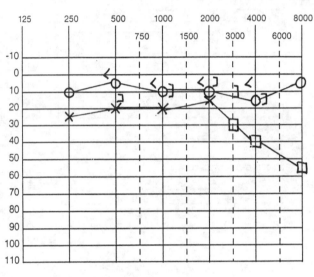

EVALUATION _____
_____
_____
_____
_____
_____
_____
_____
_____
_____
_____
_____
_____

PRACTICE CASE #7

Pt. with Alzheimer's disease. He was confused by the test situation and instructions.

MIDDLE EAR MEASURES:

	RIGHT	LEFT
ECV:	2.4 ml	2.1 ml
COMP:	.4 ml	1.2 ml
MEP:	-50 daPa	-25 daPa

Pt. Information:

M __X__ F _____ Age: __70__

SPEECH AUDIOMETRY

	SRT dB	SRT Mask	WORD RECOGNITION %	WORD RECOGNITION Mask	SL
RIGHT	40		40		30
LEFT	45		20		30
RIGHT	35	VA			
LEFT	35	VA			
BIN	35	VA	80		45

MASKING LEVELS USED

		250	500	750	1000	1500	2000	3000	4000	6000	8000
In Right (testing left)	AIR										
	BONE										
In Left (testing right)	AIR	70									
	BONE										
WEBER Lateralizes To											

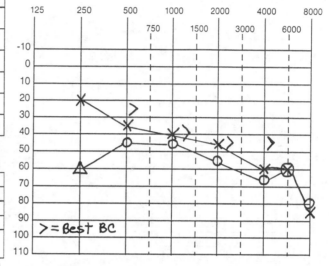

PURE-TONE AUDIOGRAM
FREQUENCY IN HERTZ (Hz)

> = Best BC

EVALUATION _____

_____
_____
_____
_____
_____
_____
_____
_____
_____
_____
_____
_____
_____

PRACTICE CASE #8

Complaint of right ear hearing loss and "itchy" ears. Right ear canal has cerumen impaction, and the left ear canal is partially obstructed.

MIDDLE EAR MEASURES:

	RIGHT	LEFT
ECV:	.4 ml	.5 ml
COMP:	0 ml	.5 ml
MEP:	Flat	0 daPa

Pt. Information:

M __X__ F _____ Age: _51_

SPEECH AUDIOMETRY

	SRT		WORD RECOGNITION		
	dB	Mask	%	Mask	SL
RIGHT	55	50	64	70	30
LEFT	20		60		30
RIGHT					
LEFT					
BIN					

MASKING LEVELS USED

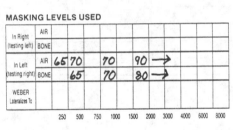

		250	500	750	1000	1500	2000	3000	4000	6000	8000
In Right (testing left)	AIR										
	BONE										
In Left (testing right)	AIR	65	70		70		90 →				
	BONE		65		70		80 →				
WEBER Lateralizes To											

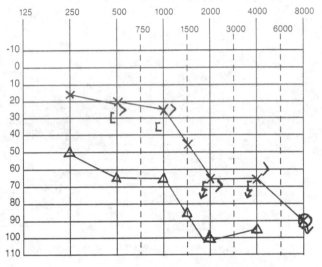

PURE-TONE AUDIOGRAM
FREQUENCY IN HERTZ (Hz)

EVALUATION _____

_____

_____

_____

_____

_____

_____

_____

_____

_____

_____

_____

_____

PRACTICE CASE #9

Hx of migrane headaches and left ear tinnitus. The CT scan is negative.

MIDDLE EAR MEASURES:	RIGHT	LEFT
ECV:	.6 ml	.7 ml
COMP:	.7 ml	.3 ml
MEP:	0 daPa	0 daPa

ACOUSTIC REFLEXES ARE ELICITED THROUGH 2000 HZ AU AND DO NOT DECAY.

Pt. Information:

M _____ F _X_ Age: _26_

SPEECH AUDIOMETRY

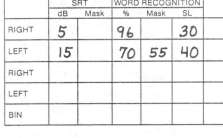

	SRT		WORD RECOGNITION		
	dB	Mask	%	Mask	SL
RIGHT	5		96		30
LEFT	15		70	55	40
RIGHT					
LEFT					
BIN					

MASKING LEVELS USED

In Right (testing left)	AIR				50	70	→		
	BONE	45	45		60	70	→		
In Left (testing right)	AIR								
	BONE								
WEBER Lateralizes To									
	250	500	750	1000	1500	2000	3000	4000	6000	8000

PURE-TONE AUDIOGRAM
FREQUENCY IN HERTZ (Hz)

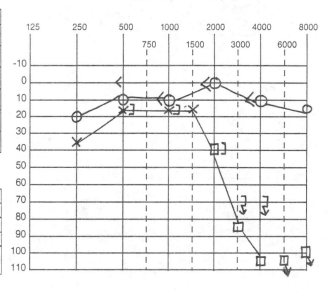

EVALUATION _____

_____

_____

_____

_____

_____

_____

_____

_____

_____

_____

PRACTICE CASE #10

Pt. sustained head injuries in MVA 3 days ago. Has basilar skull fx and bilateral hemotympanum.

MIDDLE EAR MEASURES:

	RIGHT	LEFT
ECV:	2.0 ml	2.0 ml
COMP:	.5 ml	.9 ml
MEP:	-125 daPa	-100 daPa

Pt. Information:

M __X__ F _____ Age: __22__

SPEECH AUDIOMETRY

	SRT		WORD RECOGNITION		
	dB	Mask	%	Mask	SL
RIGHT	10	45	100	50	30
LEFT	0		100	50	30
RIGHT					
LEFT					
BIN					

MASKING LEVELS USED

In Right (testing left)	AIR								
	BONE	50 →			60				
In Left (testing right)	AIR								
	BONE	50 →			60				
WEBER Lateralizes To									

250 500 750 1000 1500 2000 3000 4000 6000 8000

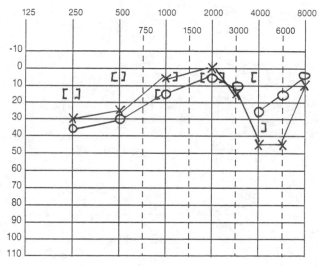

PURE-TONE AUDIOGRAM
FREQUENCY IN HERTZ (Hz)

EVALUATION

PRACTICE CASE #11

Impaired hearing since childhood. Onset attributed to gunfire. Again, as an adult, a shotgun was fired next to her. No family hx of hearing loss. No vestibular symptoms.

MIDDLE EAR MEASURES:

		RIGHT	LEFT
ECV:		.7 ml	.9 ml
COMP:		1.1 ml	1.5 ml
MEP:		-55 daPa	0 daPa

Pt. Information:

M _____ F _X_ Age: _33_

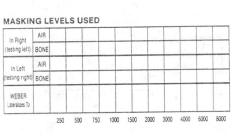

SPEECH AUDIOMETRY

	SRT		WORD RECOGNITION		
	dB	Mask	%	Mask	SL
RIGHT	20		84		35
LEFT	25		92		35
RIGHT					
LEFT					
BIN					

MASKING LEVELS USED

In Right (testing left)	AIR									
	BONE									
In Left (testing right)	AIR									
	BONE									
WEBER Lateralizes To										
		250	500	750	1000	1500	2000	3000	4000	6000	8000

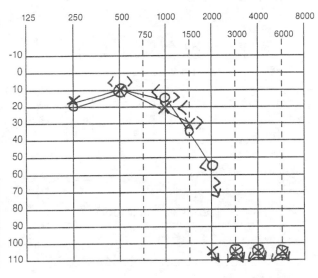

PURE-TONE AUDIOGRAM
FREQUENCY IN HERTZ (Hz)

EVALUATION

_____

_____

_____

_____

_____

_____

_____

_____

_____

_____

_____

_____

_____

PRACTICE CASE #12

Pt. was referred for medical clearance for hearing aid use. A right cholesteatoma is identified.

MIDDLE EAR MEASURES:

	RIGHT	LEFT
ECV:	1.1 ml	1.7 ml
COMP:	.1 ml	1.0 ml
MEP:	Flat	-30 daPa

Pt. Information:

M _____ F **X** Age: **54**

SPEECH AUDIOMETRY

	SRT		WORD RECOGNITION		
	dB	Mask	%	Mask	SL
RIGHT	70	60	84	80	30
LEFT	20		96		30
RIGHT					
LEFT					
BIN					

MASKING LEVELS USED

In Right (testing left)	AIR								
	BONE								
In Left (testing right)	AIR	75 →			80	90 →			
	BONE	70 →			75	80			
WEBER Lateralizes To	R	✓			✓				
		250	500	750	1000	1500	2000	3000	4000 6000 8000

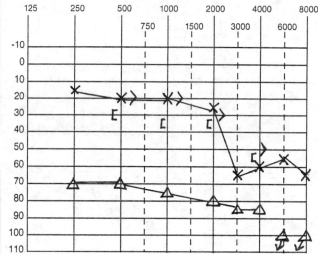

PURE-TONE AUDIOGRAM
FREQUENCY IN HERTZ (Hz)

EVALUATION _____

_____

_____

_____

_____

_____

_____

_____

_____

_____

_____

_____

_____

PRACTICE CASE #13

Hx of progressing hearing loss since young adulthood. Has worn binaural hearing aids for many years. Hearing is monitored with annual tests. Now receives little benefit from amplification.

MIDDLE EAR MEASURES:

	RIGHT	LEFT
ECV:	1.2 ml	1.7 ml
COMP:	.9 ml	1.1 ml
MEP:	0 daPa	0 daPa

Pt. Information:

M _____ F _X_ Age: _63_

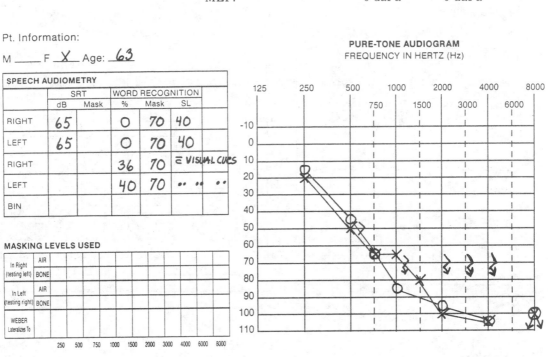

SPEECH AUDIOMETRY

	SRT		WORD RECOGNITION			
	dB	Mask	%	Mask	SL	
RIGHT	65		O	70	40	
LEFT	65		O	70	40	
RIGHT			36	70	c̄ VISUAL CUES
LEFT			40	70	•• •• ••
BIN						

MASKING LEVELS USED

		250	500	750	1000	1500	2000	3000	4000	6000	8000
In Right (testing left)	AIR										
	BONE										
In Left (testing right)	AIR										
	BONE										
WEBER Lateralizes To											

PURE-TONE AUDIOGRAM
FREQUENCY IN HERTZ (Hz)

EVALUATION _____

_____

_____

_____

_____

_____

_____

_____

_____

_____

_____

_____

_____

PRACTICE CASE #14

CC of bilateral tinnitus and hyperacusis. Hx of 44 years of blast furnace noise exposure. Does not have hearing aids.

MIDDLE EAR MEASURES:

	RIGHT	LEFT
ECV:	1.4 ml	1.0 ml
COMP:	1.3 ml	1.4 ml
MEP	-20 daPa	-30 daPa

Pt. Information:

M _X_ F _____ Age: _67_

SPEECH AUDIOMETRY

	SRT		WORD RECOGNITION		
	dB	Mask	%	Mask	SL
RIGHT	20		88		35
LEFT	20		84		35
RIGHT					
LEFT					
BIN					

MASKING LEVELS USED

In Right (testing left)	AIR									
	BONE									
In Left (testing right)	AIR									
	BONE									
WEBER Lateralizes To										
		250	500	750	1000	1500	2000	3000	4000	6000	8000

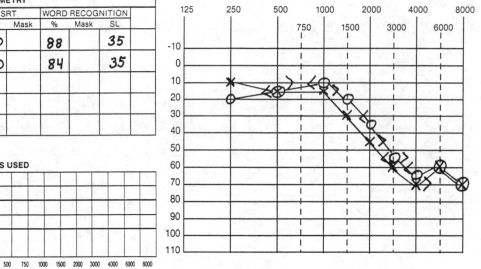

PURE-TONE AUDIOGRAM
FREQUENCY IN HERTZ (Hz)

EVALUATION _____
_____
_____
_____
_____
_____
_____
_____
_____
_____
_____
_____
_____
_____

PRACTICE CASE #15

Twenty six-year-old s/p suture ligation right ext jugular. Now with complaint of diminished hearing AD and feeling of numbness over pre-auricular area, pinna, and post-auricular area down to mandible. Also, has had frontal headache and positional dizziness since the MVA.

MIDDLE EAR MEASURES:	RIGHT	LEFT
ECV:	1.5 ml	1.4 ml
COMP:	.3 ml	.3 ml
MEP:	0 daPa	0 daPa

CONTRALATERAL AND IPSILATERAL REFLEXES ARE PRESENT AT NORMAL THRESHOLD LEVELS.

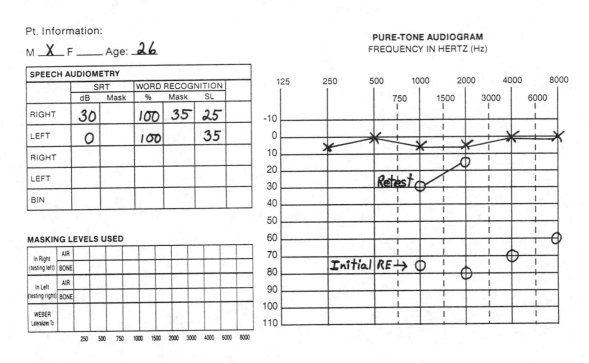

Pt. Information:

M __X__ F _____ Age: __26__

SPEECH AUDIOMETRY

	SRT		WORD RECOGNITION		
	dB	Mask	%	Mask	SL
RIGHT	30		100	35	25
LEFT	0		100		35
RIGHT					
LEFT					
BIN					

MASKING LEVELS USED

In Right (testing left)	AIR									
	BONE									
In Left (testing right)	AIR									
	BONE									
WEBER Lateralizes To										

250 500 750 1000 1500 2000 3000 4000 6000 8000

EVALUATION _____

_____

_____

_____

_____

_____

_____

_____

_____

_____

COMMONLY USED
MEDICAL ABBREVIATIONS

COMMONLY USED MEDICAL ABBREVIATIONS

A2	Aortic valve second sound
abd	Abdomen
ACTH	Adrenocorticotropic hormone
AD	Right ear
ADL	Activities of daily living
AFB	Acid fats bacilli (usually mycobacteria)
AFIB	Atrial fibrillation
AGA	Appropriate for gestational age
A/B	Albumin/globulin ratio
AKA	Above the knee amputation
AMA	Against medical advice
AML	Acute myelocytic leukemia
ANC	Absolute neutroil count
Ant	Anterior
ARDS	Acute respiratory distress syndrome
ARM	Artificial rupture of membranes
AS	Left ear
ASHD	Arteriosclerotic heart disease
AU	Both ears
AF	Atrial fibrilliation
AFL	Atrial flutter
AV	Arterviovenous
A&W	Alive and well
basco	Basophil
BBT	Basal body temperature
bHCG	Beta human chorionic gonodotrophin
bid	Twice a day (Latin: bis in dia)
BKA	Below the knee amputation
BMR	Basal metabolism rate
BPH	Benign prostatic hypertrophy
BSO	Bilaterial salpingo-oophorectomy
BSP	Bromsulphalein (a liver function test)
BTB	Break through bleeding
BUN	Blood urea nitrogen
bx	Biopsy
C&DB	Cough and deep breathe
C&S	Culture and sensitivity
Ca	Calcium
CABG	Coronary artery bypass graft
CAD	Coronary artery disease
CBC	Complete blood count
cc	Chief complaint
cc	Cubic centimeter
CHD	Coronary heart disease

CHF	Congestive heart failure
CL	Chloride
CMV	Cytomegalovirus
CNS	Central nervous system
CO2	Carbon dioxide
C/O	Complains of
coag	Coagulation
CPAP	Continuous positive airway pressure
CPR	Cardio-pulmonary resuscitation
CPT	Chest physiotherapy
CRIC	Cricoidotomy
C spine	Cervical spine
CT	Computerized axial tomography scan
CVP	Central venous pressure
CX	Axis of cylinder (ophthalmology)
cx	Cervix
CXR	Chest x-ray
D5W5%	Dextrose in water solution
D&C	Dilatation and curettage
Derm	Dermatology
diff	Differential white count
disch	Discharge
DJD	Degenerative joint disease
DOA	Dead on arrival
DOB	Date of birth
DOE	Dyspnea on exertion
DPL	Diagnostic peritoneal lavage
Dr.	Doctorp
drsg	Dressing
DT	Diptheria-tetanus toxoid
DTR	Deep tendon reflexes
dx	Diagnosis
EBL	Estimated blood loss
ECCE	Extra capsular cataract extraction
ECHO virus	Enteric cytopathogenic human orphan virus
ECT	Electroconvulsive therapy
EDC	Estimated date of confinement
EEG	Electroencephalogram
EGD	Esophago-gastro-duodenoscopy
EKG-ECG	Electrocardiogram
ENG	Electronystagmography
ENT	Ear, nose, throat
EOG	Electrooculogram

EOM	Extraocular movements
EP	Electrophysiology
ERCP	Endoscopic retrograde cholecysto pancreatogram
ERG	Electroretinogram
ET	Endotracheal
ETOH	Alcohol
EUA	Examination under anesthesia
FiO2	Oxygen concentration
FFP	Fresh frozen plasma
LFP (RFP)	Left frontoposterior (right)
LMA (RMA)	Left mentoposterior (right)
LMT (RMT)	Left mentotransverse (right)
LOP (ROP)	Left occiput posterior (right)
LOT (ROT)	Left occiput transferse (right)
LSP (RSP)	Left sacrum posterior (right)
LST (RST)	Left sacrum transverse (right)
FHR	Fetal heart rate
FHS	Fetal heart sounds
FHT	Fetal heart tones
FSH	Follicle stimuLating hormone
FTSG	Full thickness skin graft
FUO	Fever of unknown origin
fx	Fracture
Gm	Gram
GOE	gas, oxygen, ether anesthesia
gr	Grain
Grav. I	Primigravida
Grav. II	Secundigravida, etc.
GSW	Gunshot wound
GTT	Glucose tolerance test
gtt	Drop
GYN	Gynecology
Hct	Hematocrit
HCVD	Hypertensive cardiovascular disease
HEENT	Head, eyes, ears, nose, throat
HGB	Hemoglobin
HMD	Hyaline membrane disease
hs	Bedtime (Latin: hora somni)
HSG	Hystosolingogram
HNT	Hypertension
hx	History
I311	Radioactive iodine
ICU	Intensive care unit
I&D	Incision and drainage

IDM	Infant of diabetic mother
IgM	Immunoglobulin m, etc.
IMA	Internal mammary artery
IOL	Intraocular lens
IPPB	Intermittent positive pressure breathing
IVF	Intravenous fluids
IVP	Intravenous pyelogram
JVD	Jugular-venous distention
Kg	Kilogram
KUB	Kidney, ureter, bladder
L	Left
L&A	Light and accommodation
lab	Laboratory
lat	Lateral
lb	Pound
LBBB	Left bundle branch block
LDH	Lactic dehydrogenase
LLL	Left lower lobe — pulmonary
LLQ	Left lower quadrant
L/min	Liters per minute
LMP	Last menstrual period
LNMP	Last normal menstrual period
LOS	Level of consciousness
LS spine	Lumbo-sacral spine
LUL	Left upper lobe
LVH	Left ventricular hypertrophy
l&w	Living and well
lymphs	Lymphyocytes
M1	Mitral first sound
MAP	Mean arterial pressure
mcg	Microgram
mcg/dl	Microgram/deciliter
MCH	Mean corpuscular hemoglobin
MCHC	Mean corpuscular hemoglobin concentration
Meq (mEq/L)	Milliequivalents (per liter)
mg	Milligram
Mg	Magnesium
mg%	Milligrams per hundred milliliters
MHB	Maximum hospital benefit
ml	Milliliter(s) (preferred over cc)
mono	Monocyte
MRI	Magnetic resonance imaging
MRSA	Methicillin-resistant staph aureus

mv	Million volts, energy of therapeutic radiation
Na	Sodium
neuro	Neurology or neurological
NG	Naso-gastric
ng/dl	Nanograms/deciliter
NICU	Neonatal intensive care unit
NLP	No light perception
NCP	Near point of convergence
NPH	Neutral protomine hagedorn insulin
NPN	Non-protein nitrogen
NPO	Nothing by mouth (Latin: nihil per os)
NT	Nasotracheal
NWB	Non-weight bearing
O2	Oxygen
OM	Otitis media
OR	Operating room
ORIF	Open reduction and internal fixation
os	Mouth
oz	Ounce
P2	Pulmonic second heart sound
P&A	Percussion and auscultation
PA	Pulmonary artery
PAC	Premature atrial contraction
Para	# of infants born weighing 500 grams dead or alive
PAT	Paroxysmal atrial tachycardia
PBI	Protein bound iodine
PCO2	Partial pressure of carbon dioxide
Ped	Pediatric
PEG	Percutaneous endoscopic gastrostomy
PERRLA	Pupils equal, round, reactive to light and accommodation
pg/dl	Picograms/deciliter
pH	Hydrogen ion activity
PKU	Phenylketonuria
PLTS	Platelets
PMH	Past medical history
PMI	Point of maximum impulse (of heart)
PMP	Previous menstrual period
PO2	Partial pressure of oxygen
poly	Polymorphonuclear leukocyte
post op	Postoperative
PRC	Packed red cells
prep	Prepare
prn	As circumstances may require

pro time	Prothrombin time
PT	Physical therapy
PTCA	Percutaneous transluminal cardio angioplasty
PTT	Partial thromboplastin time
PWBG	Partial weight bearing
q	Every
ql	As much as desired
q. AM	Every morning
qq hor	Every hour
qd	Daily (Latin: quaque die)
qid	Four times per day (9 am - 1 pm)
qod	Every other day
q h	Every (so many) hours - q. 4h, q. 6h, etc.
R	Right
RAI	Radioactive iodine
RBBB	Right bundle branch block
RDS	Respiratory distress syndrome
Rh	Rhesus blood factor
RLF	Retrolental fibroplasia
RLL	Right lower lobe
RLQ	Right lower quandrant
RND	Radical neck dissection
R/O	Rule out
RPE	Retinal pigment epithelium
RPR	Rapid plasma reagin
R/T	Related to
RUL	Right upper lobe
RUQ	Right upper quadrant
RVH	Right ventricular hypertrophy
s	Without (Latin: sine)
SBE	Subacute bacterial endocarditis
SBO	Small bowel obstruction
sed rate	Sedimentation rate (also ESR)
SGA	Small for gestational age
SGOT	Serum glutamic oxalacetic transaminase
SGPT	Serum glutamic pyruvic transaminase
SIADH	Syndrome of inappropriate antidiuretic hormone
SLS	Sedation level score
SOB	Short of breath
SOM	Serious otitis media
Sp gr	Specific gravity
ss	A half (Latin: statim)
STSG	Split thickness skin graft

SQ	Subcutaneous
sx	Symptoms
T	Temperature
T3	Triiodethyronine
T4	Thyroxine
T&A	Tonsillectomy and adenoidectomy
T&C	Type and crossmatch
T&S	Type and screen
T spine	Thoracic spine
tab	Tablet
TAH	Total abdominal hysterectomy
Tbc	Tuberculosis
TBG	Thyroxine binding globulin
tbsp.	Tablespoon
TIA	Transient ischemic attack
tid	Three times a day
tinct	Tincture
T.O.	Telephone order
TOA	Tubal ovarian abscess
Tox	Toxicology
trach	Tracheal
TSH	Thyroid stimuLating hormone
tsp.	Teaspoon
TUR	Transurethral resection
TURP	Transurethral resection of prostate
UCG	Urinary chorionic gonadotropin
UE	Upper extremity
U/O	Urine output
URI	Upper respiratory infection
u/s	Ultrasound
UTI	Urinary tract infection
VDRL	Serology test for syphilis
vent	Ventilator
V.O.	Verbal order
VQ	Ventilation perfusion
VSD	Ventricular septal defect
Vt	Tidal volume
W&D	Warm and dry
W to d	Wet to dry
WBC	White blood count
WDWN	Well developed, well nourished
WNL	Within normal limits
XT	Exotrophia

SUGGESTED READINGS

Bess, F.H., and Humes, L.E., Eds. (1995). Audiology: The Fundamentals, Second Edition. Baltimore, MD: Williams & Wilkins.

Buckingham, R.A., Ed. (1994). Ear, Nose & Throat Diseases, A Pocket Reference, Second Edition Revised. New York, NY: Thieme.

Keith, R.W., Ed. (1981). Audiology for the Physician. Baltimore, MD: Williams & Wilkins.

Kemp, R.J., Pearson, D., & Roeser, R.J. (1995). Infection Control for the Profession of Audiology and Speech Pathology. Olathe, KS: Isles Publishers.

Lee, K.J., Ed. (1983). Essential Otolaryngology Head & Neck Surgery, Third Edition. New York, NY: Medical Exam Publishing Co.

Martin, F.N., Ed. (1981). Medical Audiology. Englewood Cliffs, NJ: Prentice-Hall.

Northern, J., Ed. (1996). Hearing Disorders, Third Edition. Needham Heights, MA: Allyn & Bacon.

Roeser, R.J. (1991). Audiology Desk Reference. New York, NY: Thieme.

Stach, B.A. (1997). Comprehensive Dictionary of Audiology. Baltimore, MD: William & Wilkins.

NOTES

NOTES

NOTES

NOTES

NOTES

NOTES

NOTES

NOTES

NOTES

NOTES